TAKE BACK YOUR HEALTH

TAKE BACK YOUR HEALTH

✦

A TOTAL WELLNESS GUIDE FOR YOU AND YOUR FAMILY

Renee A. Simon, M.S., C.N.S.
Board Certified Clinical Nutritionist

Foreword by Michael Finkelstein, M.D.

iUniverse, Inc.
New York Lincoln Shanghai

TAKE BACK YOUR HEALTH
A TOTAL WELLNESS GUIDE FOR YOU AND YOUR FAMILY

iUniverse books may be ordered through booksellers or by contacting:

iUniverse
2021 Pine Lake Road, Suite 100
Lincoln, NE 68512
www.iuniverse.com
1-800-Authors (1-800-288-4677)

The information in this book is for educational purposes only and is not recommended as a means of diagnosing or treating an illness. Please consult a medical or other professional if you have questions about your health. The statements about the food supplements have not been evaluated by the Food & Drug Administration.

ISBN-13: 978-0-595-34891-6 (pbk)
ISBN-13: 978-0-595-79609-0 (ebk)
ISBN-10: 0-595-34891-2 (pbk)
ISBN-10: 0-595-79609-5 (ebk)

Printed in the United States of America

Long Before....

Processed, Super Sized Meals, Over Prescribed Drugs & Sedentary & Stressful Lifestyles

....There was Optimal Health

To all of you who want to maximize your energy and vitality and take your health to a new level

I ask everyone here to continue your prayers and vigils on behalf of the Long Lost Boat.

Contents

Part III   Anti-Aging Program for Energy & Vitality

Acknowledgments

I would like to thank all of the editors and reviewers who have helped me to get this book to you. Special thanks to Dr. Michael Finkelstein, Tish Tamowski, Cheryl Fish, Brenda Bergstrom, Doris Henderson, Peter Howland, and Dr. David Brady. I would also like to thank Truus Teeuwissen for doing a fine job on the book cover on such short notice.

Special gratitude goes to all of my patients who have confirmed my belief that if you nourish the body with proper food, rest, nutrients, exercise and stress relief, incredible healing takes place.

Lastly, I would like to thank my parents, Lila and George Fish for their everlasting love and support.

Foreword

One of the remarkable issues I observe as a physician in today's world is the paradox between the number of self help books and gurus and the number of truly healthy people. While it could be said that the interest in such material is proportional to the need, I see it differently; I believe there is something lacking from the messages touted by most, especially the particularly popular ones that seem to surface every five to ten years. More so, their books often outline plans that mislead individuals into thinking that the process is easy. And finally, they are all too often geared toward narrowly focused goals, particularly weight loss.

It is refreshing to read a book written by someone who herself has gone through the painful and slow learning curve who leads us to a greater understanding of the process itself. In this book, Renee Simon, recounts with unabashed honesty how she came to realize what "wellness" is. And she further states, with humility, that each of us needs to identify that for one's self. Then, does she first begin to suggest how we might approach such an understanding. This is not a program that is "one size fits all."

Instead, through the illustrations of real patients, she shows us how one pieces together an individual plan that combines nutrition with other lifestyle adjustments. Her background is scientific, but she is not limited by the Western medical paradigm. Thus, her approach is more complete and takes into account emotional, spiritual and the connectedness of all of these things as part of the whole.

It is very likely that you will lose weight if you follow Renee's sound advice and reasoning, if that is your primary objective. But this book is much more than that. As I read through it, I imagined what individuals in my own family reading this book would get out of it—my mother one thing, my father, wife, and children something else. It is applicable for all of them and perhaps most compelling is the notion that they would all read it and be able to come together to help each other with the necessary modifications.

This book is aptly titled "Take Back Your Health" because that is what it describes—the journey for a better self. The results for many of its readers will be an eye-opening revelation. The concept of "Total Wellness" addresses what each of us in our core is likely to find: a desire to be lighter and healthier. This is obviously more than a literal reference and those who read on and, most importantly, those who make use of its recommendations will be rewarded to find how tangible this is.

Michael B. Finkelstein, M.D., F.A.C.P.
Center for Health and Healing of Northern Westchester
Mount Kisco, NY
March 2005

Introduction

Lila and Georges's second child was a happy, playful girl until age five, when her behavior suddenly changed. Temper tantrums, wall kicking, and moodiness seemed to take over her previously cheerful personality. After seeing many doctors, the child was diagnosed with allergies and began a treatment program that included allergy shots, nose sprays, antihistamines, frequent use of antibiotics, and occasional use of steroids. While this program helped with some of her symptoms initially, none of the doctors ever advised the family to stop the medication. She continued with the prescribed program until she was 25 years old.

That little girl was me. I am now 43. As an adult I have had many of the health issues (Epstein Barr virus, food sensitivities, hypoglycemia, digestive problems, infertility, interstitial cystitis, and hormonal imbalances) that are described in this book.

Was it a coincidence that I had poor health in my 20's and 30's, or was it the overuse of allergy medicine and antibiotics? My theory is that the long-term medical treatment weakened my immune, digestive and reproductive systems, with stress and environmental factors as the final ingredients that made me sick.

How many Americans like me have been over-medicated, their care miss-managed as they were passed from doctor to doctor? With all this compounded by poor diets, environmental toxins, and stress, it is easy to see why we are in a health crisis.

Two thirds of our adults are either overweight or obese. Add to that equation the large number of people with diabetes and high blood pressure. It is clear that many people are walking time bombs for heart disease, the number one killer in the U.S. In addition, more than 20 million couples have been diagnosed with infertility. Men and women are popping pills daily for reflux, depression, headaches, asthma, allergies, arthritis, and other chronic conditions.

Our children have a health crisis too. Among kids between six and 19 years old, one in six is overweight. One in 250 children is now diagnosed with autism or a related disorder, and more than two million are estimated to have Attention Deficit Disorder (ADD) or Attention Deficit Hyperactivity Disorder (ADHD).

What do all of these problems have in common? To a significant extent they are based on nutritional deficiencies and metabolic imbalances that can be helped using my proven four-step program that combines clinical testing with dietary interventions, vitamin and mineral therapies, exercise recommendations, and stress management techniques.

My motivation for writing this book is to help you reclaim your health and vitality, which will help you take better care of everyone else who is important to you. As women, we tend to neglect ourselves. My patients frequently do whatever it takes to help their children, spouses or parents, but when it comes to their own needs they fall short. They often work long hours at an outside job or at home and then cart the kids around to a long list of activities to ensure there is enough physical and intellectual stimulation. Some of my patients who have picky eaters may cook two to three entrees at each meal, only to pick at food throughout the day themselves and never sit down to a balanced meal.

While self-help books exist on many of the individual topics covered in *Take Back Your Health*, I wanted to give you one place to look to help everyone that you care about using an easy to read format. My objective is for you to use this book as a resource for your entire family. For instance, you may pick up this book because you are experiencing fatigue or gastric reflux. After following the recommendations and feeling better you might want to pass it along to your spouse for high cholesterol, your mother for diabetes, or to your niece who has asthma.

This book is an account of my experiences in nutrition for close to a decade. First I describe my personal journey recovering from illnesses physically, emotionally and spiritually. Then through patient make-over examples, I will show you how to use dietary interventions, vitamin and mineral therapies, and exercise and stress management programs to help you with common medical conditions. The names of the people in the makeover examples and some of the identifying information have been changed in all cases to ensure anonymity.

The main part of the book is divided into five sections:

Section 1: Protect Your Heart—Which covers how to lose weight, improve cholesterol and triglycerides, decrease hypertension, balance blood sugar, and prevent or reverse diabetes. This section has two makeover examples to show you how you can make practical changes to your diet and life style to achieve better health.

Section 2: Balance Hormones Naturally—Which covers how to boost fertility, heal PMS, and have a smooth perimenopause to menopause transition. This section has four makeover examples to show you how to balance your hormones and reach your objectives whether that means getting pregnant or getting rid of PMS, interstitial cystitis, or menopause symptoms.

Section 3: Improve Your Digestive Health—Which covers how to help crohn's, colitis, irritable bowel, diarrhea, constipation, gas, bloating, and gastric reflux using a 4-R recovery program to <u>remove</u> toxic substances, <u>replace</u> them with good nutrition, <u>reintroduce</u> enzymes and probiotics, and finally <u>repair</u> the gut with vitamins, minerals, and amino acids. This section has three makeover examples that illustrate how others have naturally helped these problems in addition to improving their allergies, asthma, and psoriasis once their digestive issues were resolved.

Section 4: Enhance Your Children's Health—Help without drugs for allergies, asthma, ear infections, ADD/ADHD, autism, sensory, immune, and digestive problems. The three makeover examples reveal the most important tests to detect nutritional deficiencies and how to modify the diet and use supplements to improve biochemical balance. These programs even work for picky eaters.

Section 5: The final section of the book outlines an anti-aging program just for you. This section covers how to have more energy, maintain optimal weight, look and feel youthful, and prepare for a lifetime of health with vitality.

I have included my story and the experiences of others to help you find information that will assist you and your family in your own health and healing journey. I want to send thanks to my patients whose stories are reflected in these pages and to all of the others whom I am privileged to have served. Thank you for helping me spread the message of preventative and restorative health.

Yours in good health,
Renee Simon

PART I
My Personal Journey

1

Health Crisis & Recovery

I often wonder where my life would be now if I hadn't developed the Epstein Barr* virus out of the blue eleven years ago. Would I still be in a thankless, stressful job striving to make the next promotion? Would I be childless, missing one of the most rewarding aspects of my life? Would I be following the standard American diet, oblivious to the needs of my body?

When you are sick it is hard to look at the good it brings when you are in the crux of it. But as many who have gone through the process know, it can bring about incredible change, often positive and life-altering.

That is what happened to me. Prior to May of 1992, I was healthy (or so I thought) and reasonably content, although much of it was tied to the material wealth I had accumulated. What I didn't realize at the time was how unbalanced my life really was. Most of my time was spent working or thinking about work. The little free time I had was spent running; I often ran 20-30 miles a week. I was literally on a treadmill all of the time, always running, driving hard, striving to get ahead. I didn't realize that my body was experiencing classic adrenal stress burnout,* always in fight or flight mode. This was taking an enormous toll on my overall physical health and preparing me for an immune system crash.

---

*   (NOTE: Any terms marked by an asterisk (*) indicate their inclusion in the glossary)

Why Me, Why Now?

Was it my stressful job that made me sick? Clearly it was a factor, but not the only one. I attribute my illness to a series of events that happened over the first thirty years of my life. To begin, I was a sickly child with bad allergies. I was given allergy shots for irritants from the time I was five until I was 25 years old. No one ever told me that such long-term treatment might have a negative effect on my liver or my immune system. In addition, I was always using antihistamines, nose sprays, antibiotics, or steroids when things got really bad. Little by little, my immune system was being assaulted, and without proper nutrition, I was getting beat.

Added to that, at the age of 15, I got into a bad car accident that almost killed me. The car hit an embankment, caught fire, and turned over. Friends in a car right next to ours pulled us to safety and had the ambulance over in a matter of minutes. Nevertheless, I found myself in the hospital with a severe compound fracture of my left arm, a concussion, and lacerations on the left side of my body. I was clearly lucky to be alive but in need of surgery and high doses of antibiotics to help with infections before they could even operate.

I recovered well from the surgery and had to get another operation a year later to take out the pins and plates that were holding my left arm together.

Was That All?

I wish I could say that was the end of hospital visits and trips to the doctor. About twelve years later I started my infertility roller coaster. It really wasn't a surprise because I was diagnosed with endometriosis about two years prior after having a laparotomy* and a large cyst the size of an orange removed from my ovary. Endometriosis is a common condition that occurs when the endometrial lining attaches to the ovaries, uterus or parts of the abdominal cavity and pelvis instead of completely shedding every month during menstruation. This causes painful periods, bloating, and inflammation. Not only was my immune system failing, but my endocrine system as well.

After years of painful periods I was relieved to find out what was wrong. I wasn't prepared for the six surgeries that followed each time the endometriosis came back or the drug therapy that made me gain 15 pounds, grow facial hair, and be an irritable mess. Nor was I prepared to be an emotional basket case each time someone in the family gave birth and relatives would say, "Why don't you start a family?"

What Role Does Unhappiness and Sadness Play?

It was not only the physical wear and tear on my body that the infertility treatments and surgeries caused, but the constant sadness and lack of emotional support during this difficult time that contributed to my physical and mental distress. Even though I was married, my husband didn't care if we had a baby, which put the entire burden of the treatments on me without a compatriot to share the living hell that it was. Sadness, unhappiness, living without support can cause emotional conflict which can manifest unconsciously in the physical body and trigger a variety of energy imbalances and physical symptoms. Had I known better I would have practiced yoga, meditation, visualization exercises, or tai chi to help heal my body and calm my spirit, but it would be years before my holistic awakening occurred.

Health Crisis

After years of infertility treatments and job stress that found me looking at a job in Cincinnati, far away from friends and family, I woke up one morning with the worst sore throat I ever had, large swollen glands, and fatigue that barely allowed me to get out of bed.

Thinking I had strep throat, I went to my neighborhood physician for antibiotics. He told me the culture was negative yet I didn't get any better after a week. I started to worry. After weeks of a low-grade fever, foggy brain, malaise, and debilitating fatigue I went in for blood work.

The good news was that I was diagnosed early with active Epstein Barr virus titers* that were off the charts. For some people it takes years to get a definitive diagnosis, even though they are obviously sick. For years Epstein Barr Virus and Chronic Fatigue Syndrome, a disorder that is related in some cases, were dismissed by many doctors as diseases for women who were hypochondriacs or who had emotional problems. Luckily that was not my case. The bad news, however, was that no medical treatments existed besides rest. I was too proud to admit to my boss that I was sick, which made a medical leave of absence out of the question, so I found myself going from doctor to doctor looking for a cure.

The Cure was Slow to Find, but Quick to Work

For the first time in my life, conventional medicine could not help me. I realized I needed to explore the physical, emotional, and spiritual aspects of my illness from a holistic perspective before any healing could take place. Even though I had no experience in holistic health at this time, my intuition led me to a naturopathic physician, a holistic medical doctor, and a library of research to explore what alternatives were available to jump start my immune system to bring my body into balance.

The naturopath was convinced that a large part of my problem was caused by poor digestive function leading to food allergies. He tested me for allergies and nutritional imbalances using a machine that monitors energy levels according to the body's meridians* and shows imbalances that exist. The results of the tests showed sensitivities to almost everything I was eating. As a result, I completely eliminated sugar, caffeine, alcohol, and junk foods from my diet and ate brown rice, organic fruits and vegetables, and proteins like turkey, eggs, and fish. I even did a water fast for awhile to detoxify my body and then juiced fruits and vegetables to maximize my vitamin and mineral intake. In addition, the naturopath made drops for me to take under my tongue of minute quantities of the things that I was sensitive to in order to build up an immunity to those substances over time.

The holistic medical doctor that I was seeing specialized in using intravenous vitamin and chelation treatments to help patients with heart disease, cancer and immune system problems. I was given an IV with 75 grams of vitamin C as well as other minerals I was low in. I was also put on mega-doses of oral nutrients to boost my immune system and improve my energy.

Although I kept working during this time, my hours were reduced and I took a 30 day vacation to regroup and work on the emotional and spiritual aspects of my disease. There were many things about myself and the person that I had become that I wasn't proud of. Meditation and visualization exercises, seeing myself as a healthier, kinder person, became part of my daily routine. During these explorations, my corporate job became meaningless. I imagined a life of service to others incorporating everything I learned during my recovery. I wanted to broaden my spiritual side and become more connected to nature and the larger world outside of myself. As renowned psychologist Dr. Maslow said, I was becoming "self-actualized" on my spiritual journey.

My Recovery/Awakening

After four months of holistic medical treatments and my own research and self-discovery I was starting to get better. I often tell the patients that I see that recovery is a slow process. An illness takes many years to manifest, so reversing the process can take many years as well. It's like peeling back layers of physical and emotional baggage that brought on the disease; to get better, one layer at a time must be healed. Sorry to say, there are no magic pills or instant cures. The dietary changes and supplements were helping me physically, and through journaling, meditating, and visualizing I was slowly healing my inner spirit and physical core. Yet, there was something missing to tip my health into the recovered column. I link this to the sadness that I spoke of earlier and the emptiness that I felt having not been successful in getting pregnant.

Eleven months after the start of my illness my husband and I got a call that we were to be adoptive parents. A birthmother had selected us to be the parents of her unborn child. We had submitted the paperwork months before. Now I had a true reason to get better—there was a child who needed me.

The bit of elation and the subsequent preparation that focused on something other than my illness was what it took to tip that scale over to recovery. That was January of 1993; our daughter was born in April of that year, a beautiful answer to my prayers.

Using What I Learned to Change My Life

After our daughter was born I took six months off from work and immersed myself into motherhood. We went on daily walks, did the mommy and me classes and with what little free time a new mom has I thought of ways to change my career and life to a more fulfilling one. I wanted to use my experiences to help others recover or better yet, to teach people to avoid the disease process to begin with and live a healthy and happy life.

Over the next few years, I reduced the time at my corporate job and eventually left altogether to pursue a master's degree in clinical nutrition. Clinical nutrition involves finding underlying causes of sickness and disease to bring the body into balance through dietary recommendations, vitamin, mineral, and herbal therapies, and stress management techniques—the same steps that I followed to get well again.

After graduation, I worked closely with a Developmental Pediatrician who specialized in holistic treatments for children with special needs such as Attention Deficit Hyperactivity Disorder (ADHD),* Autistic Spectrum Disorder (ASD),* Pervasive Developmental Disorder (PDD),* Sensory Integration Dysfunction (SID),* and Down 's syndrome. I loved working with children, but after several years decided to expand my practice to work with entire families.

Physical, Emotional, and Spiritual Lessons Learned

There are so many things that I learned from my illness that I would like to share with you. First, healing is an ongoing journey. When you solve one physical or emotional problem there is always more to look at. This does not mean dwelling on illness or solving problems that do not exist. It simply means uncovering emotional, spiritual, and physical layers that need to be looked at on a regular basis.

Second, take responsibility for your own health and wellness. If you are sick, surround yourself with the best that eastern and western medicine offers. But don't rely solely on your doctors and natural practitioners to get you well. You must research, look into your body, trust your instincts, and put the best integrated program together for yourself. The key is to never give up. If one thing doesn't work, try something else.

Third, don't believe what people tell you about recovery time. I was told it would take years to get better or that I never would. I remember going to a support group meeting and seeing people who were debilitated for years with Chronic Fatigue Syndrome. I never went back because I didn't want any preconceived notions in my head about how long my recovery would take.

Fourth, you need support. Although support group meetings aren't for everyone, it is important to have people in your life that are supportive. There is evidence that loving support and prayer can be crucial to get over or live successfully with an illness.

Fifth, take a step back and evaluate what you can learn from your experience. When in the middle of an illness or difficult time in your life, find out why this is happening now, and what can be learned from your experience. I am a firm believer that most things in life happen for a reason. In my case, I was being told to slow down and take stock of my life. It could mean taking time to heal an old wound or facing something that you have been putting off.

Sixth, find something larger than yourself to think and care about. When you are sick it is so easy to be all consumed by the illness. Being there and doing for others is sometimes the best medicine of all.

Lastly, don't compare yourself to anyone else on your road to recovery. Some people can eat what they want and never get sick, and others have to take very good care of themselves to stay healthy. The key is to know who you are and what your body needs.

In addition, there are several key steps that I followed to help my recovery which are also reflected in the patient makeovers throughout this book, and are the same steps that I recommend you look at when creating your own Total Wellness program. While the steps are the same, the actual components of each step will be different based on individual needs.

The Following is a summary of my total wellness makeover:

Before Illness

Diet:	Mostly vegetarian—eating mixed grains, fruits and vegetables, with eggs, cheese, and fish for protein. I consumed two-three cups of coffee a day with cookies, candy, chips, soda, and cake when they were available. I drank a lot of water and also consumed some diet soda and juice. Consumed two-three alcoholic beverages on the week-end.
Supplements:	Basic multiple vitamin and vitamin C. Occasionally took echinacea when I had a cold.
Exercise:	Was training for a marathon and ran about 35-40 miles per week. Occasionally worked out with weights.
Stress Mgt. & Self-Care:	Very little. Worked long hours at corporate job. Took work home on week-ends. Volunteered as a Big Sister. Periodically wrote in journal.

Recovery Program after Illness

Diet:	Cut down starches to non-allergic ones: brown rice, and yams. Ate only organic fruits and vegetables. Consumed a variety of grain fed meat (mostly lamb and venison), fish, eggs, and poultry. Added nuts, and legumes such as soy, garbanzo, and black beans. My fats were restricted to olive, flax, and canola oils. Ate no junk food initially. Did not consume any sugar other than fruit for over two years. Eliminated caffeine and alcohol. Drank water and herbal teas only.
Supplements:	For three months I did IV vitamins with a high dose of vitamin C. As I improved I could absorb oral supplements and took a multi-vitamin and mineral complex, vitamins C, E, B, zinc, selenium, CoQ10, calcium, magnesium, and L-Carnitine.
Exercise:	Had to cut my exercise down substantially. Walked two-three days per week as I could tolerate it. As my energy improved I began to add five minutes more each time. I also added stretching and yoga.
Stress Mgt. & Self-Care:	Practiced mindful meditation and trying to live in the moment even when I wasn't feeling very well. Did daily visualization exercises, seeing myself healthy doing the kinds of things I wanted to do again. Cut back my work schedule. Wrote in my journal daily.

Step 1: Diet

After my food and nutrient testing, it was clear that I was sensitive to many foods, particularly dairy and wheat products. As a result, I reduced my grain intake to brown rice and also consumed white potatoes and yams in moderation. The rest of my diet consisted of organic fruits and vegetables, grain fed organic lamb and turkey, eggs, beans, nuts, and fish. My fats were restricted to olive, flax, almond, and fish oils. All of the extras were cut out of my diet and for awhile water and herbal teas were my only beverages. While this diet may seem very restrictive, it is actually quite healthy and hypo-allergenic for those who suspect food sensitivities. It can be followed for a short time as you cleanse your system of foods that can't be tolerated, or long-term for a life time of good health.

Step 2: Exercise

Because of my illness I could no longer run. This was very difficult for me. Epstein Barr Virus is an example of an illness where expending high degrees of energy or being too physically active before you are ready can cause major setbacks. As I gradually felt better, I was able to walk aerobically, adding more mileage each week. I also added stretching and yoga to my program.

Step 3: Supplements

My supplement level was very high initially. Intravenous nutrient therapy is usually used when the digestive tract can not properly digest vitamins and minerals from food or supplements or when the doses are so high they need to be administered with a slow drip to avoid negative side effects. As I got better, I was able to tolerate oral supplements and took a multi-vitamin and mineral complex, vitamins C, E, B complex, zinc, selenium, CoQ10,* calcium, magnesium, and L-Carnitine.*

Step 4: Stress Management & Self-Care

I also made sure to find pleasure and joy each day, even when I felt sick or depressed. I appreciated flowers or trees outside, read good books, and laughed watching old "I Love Lucy" reruns. It's sometimes these small little bits of joy or laughter accumulated every day that can be the missing ingredient to recovery.

Meditation and visualization exercises became part of my daily routine. Meditation was a stress reducer and gave me insight into the healing process. Visualization exercises allowed me to see myself healthy, doing the kinds of things that I enjoy.

Enough said about my personal journey. The next section of the book will discuss common illnesses and what to do about them using many of my patient case histories.

PART II

Total Wellness Makeovers for You & the People You Care About

2

Protect Your Heart

In the recent documentary *Super Size Me,* filmmaker Morgan Spurlock proves the dangers of fast food by going on a 30 day binge of eating nothing but McDonald's. His goal is to educate Americans about the dangers of fast food and the highly processed diet. The film highlights the problems with the food in the school systems which are largely fast food, pre-cooked meals and vending machine based, driven by school incentive programs.

Spurlock points out that in the last 25 years there has been a doubling of childhood obesity and predicts if the trend continues one out of three children will develop diabetes during their lifetime. He also blames the food industry lobbyists and companies who target children early with mega-advertising of fast foods. In one comical scene in the movie he asked children of different age groups to identify pictures of America's founding fathers. While many of them cannot identify George Washington and do not know anything about Abraham Lincoln, they all can identify Ronald McDonald and sing many of the fast food jingles.

At the end of the movie, doctors reveal the results of Morgan's fast food makeover: his weight went from 185-210, his cholesterol from 168 to 225, his body fat from 11 to 18%, liver enzymes elevated to dangerous levels suggesting fatty liver disease, and finally his uric acid levels elevated, suggesting he was prone to getting gout and kidney disease.

The take home message from the movie was clearly to limit the amount of fast and processed foods you consume and feed your children. It is important to start your family on a healthy path as early in life as possible, including 30 minutes of exercise a day, and a balanced fresh-food diet. Hopefully that will start to have an impact on the 400,000 deaths per year related to obesity and its associated diseases.

Syndrome X, or Metabolic Syndrome, are terms coined by the medical community to mean a cluster of risk factors that are interrelated and tied to obesity. They can lead to a variety of life threatening diseases. It is thought that as many as 40-50 % of Americans over 50 have some or all of the characteristics of this disorder. The most common characteristics are:

Elevated fasting and non fasting insulin levels
Elevated fasting glucose
High triglycerides (over 100 mg/dl)
High low-density lipoprotein (LDL)—bad cholesterol more than 100 mg/dl
Low high-density lipoprotein (HDL)—good cholesterol under 45 mg/dl
Hypertension—blood pressure over 115/75 mm Hg
Waist circumference > 35 inches for women; and > 40 inches for men
Body Mass Index (BMI) over 30
To calculate your BMI use the formula: BMI = (weight in pounds/height in inches^2) x 703. For example, a person who weighs 128 and is 5 feet 4 inches tall has a BMI of 21.97: (128 lbs/ 64^2) X 703 = 21.97.

The diseases that are often associated with this disorder are type II diabetes, coronary heart disease, systemic inflammation, degenerative arthritis, and cancer (endometrial and breast for women and prostrate and colon for men). According to a March 2004 *Time Magazine* article entitled "Inflammation, the Secret Killer," inflammation is now thought to be one of the common threads in all of the diseases listed above. Inflammatory stimuli, such as bacterial infections, trauma, ischemic events, stress-related events, toxic exposures, allergens, and chronic viral infections, all activate the inflammatory response and can be causative factors.

This syndrome is not something that happens in one day. It evolves over years by living an unhealthy life style. It relates back to the industrialization of America and the change from eating fresh, hand picked food off the farm to eating what has become the standard American diet. Instead of choosing whole fruits and vegetables, fresh grains and meats, we began eating highly processed foods filled with unnatural fats, artificial sweeteners, pesticides, preservatives, and chemicals. Instead of walking, we found it more convenient driving in our cars. Instead of playing outside after school, children began watching non-stop television and using computers. It relates to our convenience and quick fix mentality.

We take prepared foods out of a package or fast food restaurant, pop our meals in the microwave, and eat as quickly as we can while watching our favorite television show. Then we go to the refrigerator/freezer and pull out a chocolate bar, some ice cream, or bottle of wine to drown out our feelings of anger, sadness, or unfulfilled dreams or to reward ourselves for making it through another grueling day.

After consuming a diet high in sugar and refined carbohydrates for many years, the pancreas malfunctions and can no longer control the amount of insulin needed to process glucose (blood sugar). This creates a condition known as insulin resistance, which simply means too much insulin in the blood. It often goes hand in hand with weight gain, cholesterol elevation, high blood pressure, and diabetes.

According to National Health and Nutrition Examination Survey (NHANES) data, approximately 67% of American adults are either overweight (characterized by a BMI over 25) or obese (BMI over 30) and 15% of children are overweight. Metabolic and insulin resistance syndromes start years before diabetes, cardiovascular disease, or cancer develops.

Many people feel that their illnesses are the outcome of flawed genes. They look for the magic pill to fix the problem. Although genes play an important role in the risk of disease, there are many things you can do to change the result. The growing field of "nutrigenomics" is teaching people to use nutrition (diet and supplements) to improve gene outcomes. The science of nutrigenomics is the study of how naturally occurring chemicals in foods alter molecular expression of genetic information in each individual. I heard a metaphor recently that describes this pretty well. Your genes act like a loaded gun that you carry around with you. It is up to you, through your dietary and life style habits, to pull the trigger or not.

People are now living much longer. If you expect to live with health for ten decades you have to go beyond your genes to take care of yourself. That means you must change your habits **NOW** to prevent these diseases. If someone you care about already has some of the risk factors we mentioned, you can help them reverse the process. The keys are diet, weight loss, exercise, nutritional supplements along with stress management and self-care techniques. The following are some makeover examples to help you through the process.

Brian's Health Makeover—Overweight, High Cholesterol & Triglycerides, Osteoarthritis

Background

Brian was a retired 60 year old who came to see me to lose weight and lower his cholesterol and triglycerides. He was on medication for high triglycerides and blood pressure. His starting weight was 240 in a 6'2" frame. His body mass index was about 31, which put him just in the obese range.

During the first few appointments I analyzed Brian's diet and found he was eating too many refined carbohydrates like pretzels and cookies as snacks throughout the day to keep his energy up. He was starting the day with a sugary low-fiber cereal that was setting him up to be hungry and tired in about an hour. Sugary foods (considered high glycemic*) cause a quick rise in blood sugar followed by a surge in insulin which drives the blood sugar down fast. It is much healthier to eat low glycemic, high fiber carbohydrates, which create a gradual rise in blood sugar and insulin and a gradual fall. That way energy is balanced and food cravings and hunger are managed.

Brian was eating sandwiches for lunch, usually followed by pretzels and cookies and an occasional fruit. For dinner he consumed large portions of protein and starch with a small side of vegetables. Sometimes there were a few more cookies after dinner or another dessert.

Over the years Brian's exercise level had decreased since he had experienced some knee and shoulder injuries.

Treatment

Diet

I educated Brian about eating the right carbohydrates—low glycemic, high fiber—and healthy snacks with a balance of some protein and fiber. Examples are a handful of almonds, low-fat cheese with whole grain crackers, or apple slices with natural peanut butter. We also discussed portion control with his dinner meal.

In addition, I asked Brian to switch to egg white omelettes with vegetables a couple of mornings a week, and salads with fish, turkey, chicken, or low-fat cheese for lunch instead of sandwiches, to cut down on the amount of carbohydrates he consumed. While farmed salmon and albacore tuna are high in the good omega-3 fatty acids, they also tend to be high in health-threatening toxins. These should be limited to no more than once or twice a month. Sole, cod, flounder, haddock, red snapper, halibut, and bluefish might have half as many essential fatty acids, but they have much lower toxin levels.

Supplements

I introduced several supplements to help bring down Brian's cholesterol and triglyceride levels which also helped him to continue to lose weight without hitting a plateau.

I recommended a fiber supplement made of psyllium husk and other soluble fiber* to help pull cholesterol out of his body and to aid in weight loss. Taking fiber with a large glass of water before meals helps the person fill up so they are less starved during the meal. I also added fish oil (EPA/DHA)* which helps to lower cholesterol and triglycerides, keeps the blood clean with less arterial plaque, and L-Carnitine, a natural fat burner—good for cholesterol and triglyceride management, overall cellular energy, and heart health. Other supplements for general health and energy metabolism were a multi-vitamin and mineral complex, B-complex, and Calcium/Magnesium for the aches and pains he was experiencing. Brian later added glucosamine sulfate* and manganese to help with his joint problems.

Exercise

With a little help from the chiropractor that I referred him to, who worked on his knee and shoulder injuries, Brian was able to start an exercise program. It consisted of walking with his dogs one to two miles, three times per week. He also added light weight lifting, which helped his knee and shoulder.

Results

After the first six weeks on the diet Brian lost 15 lbs. He felt much better than he had in years. His energy was higher throughout the day, and he was more alert, with better concentration.

After another few weeks Brian had his blood lipid panel checked. He was amazed at how much his numbers had improved. His total cholesterol went from 260 to 205, his HDL went from 39 to 49, and his LDL from 165 to 135. The most impressive change was his triglycerides, which went from 279 to 105. Brian stated that in 25 years his triglycerides were never normal. His walking was now increased to 1 mile a day with some light running mixed in. At our last meeting, about 8 months after he started his program, Brian was down to 200, with his goal weight of 195, and BMI of 25 in sight.

Summary

What worked for Brian was slow steady progress in weight loss and quick improvements in how he felt. With more energy and fewer joint problems, Brian was able to greatly increase his exercise, which helped with his lipid profile, weight management and sense of well-being. He didn't feel that he was really giving up much in his diet. Once in awhile he can eat an occasional snack food without any trouble. He no longer cares to eat the quick fix carbohydrates because he feels much better without them. In fact, he doesn't find himself craving foods nearly as much.

Brian's case illustrates that with the right program begun early enough, many of the characteristics of syndrome X can be reversed, and disorders like heart disease and osteoarthritis can be avoided. Unlike rheumatoid arthritis, an autoimmune disease that can affect people of all ages, osteoarthritis is a common degenerative disease resulting from years of joint usage that can be improved with proper nutrition, weight loss and supplements.

Brian's Makeover: Before

Diet:	Lot's of refined carbohydrates including white bread, pretzels, sugary cereals, and cookies. Portions of pasta and protein were too high. Not enough fruits, whole grain, legumes, and vegetables.
Weight/Cholesterol:	Brian's starting weight was 240, height 6'2, BMI =31. Cholesterol: 260.
Triglycerides:	Triglycerides: 279.
Supplements:	Brian was not taking any to start.

Exercise:	Brian was limited by osteoarthritis in his knee and shoulder. He walked a little but was not able to sustain a balanced exercise program.
Stress Mgt. & Self-Care:	This was not really something Brian thought about. He was semi-retired and did not think he was under a lot of stress. He didn't really understand the mind-body connection and the effect of stress on obesity.

Brian's Makeover: After Total Wellness Program

Diet:	Balanced diet using 40/30/30 principles. All carbohydrates consumed are low glycemic and high fiber. Portion sizes are moderate for grains and protein. Fruits, vegetables, whole grain, and legumes as well as healthy fats and quality protein now make up the majority of Brian's diet.
Weight/Cholesterol:	Brian's weight was reduced to 200 after 6 months, height 6'2, BMI =25.7. Cholesterol: 205.
Triglycerides:	Triglycerides: 105.
Supplements:	Brian started taking a fiber supplement to help with his cholesterol. He also added fish oil, L-Carnitine, a multi-vitamin, B-complex, calcium/magnesium, glucosamine sulfate, and manganese for his osteoarthritis.
Exercise:	Once his arthritis improved, Brian was able to walk one to two miles every day and add in some light running. He also started a weight lifting program to continue to improve his knee and shoulder.
Stress Mgt. & Self-Care:	Although it is hard to teach an old dog new tricks, Brian realized that his daily stresses did impact his health and outlook on life. Even though he wasn't interested in taking up yoga or learning how to meditate, he was open to listening more to his body and making sure to spend quality time every day doing one or two activities he enjoyed.

Carol's Health Makeover—Weight Loss, Allergies, Sinus and Yeast Infections

Background

Carol was 40 when she came to see me. She was 5'4" and weighed 245 lbs. She had gained a lot of weight with her three pregnancies and was never able to get back to her pre-pregnancy weight of 150. She wanted a program that would allow slow, gradual weight loss, help boost her energy level, and provide a healthy eating program for her whole family, who were all overweight.

Carol worked long hours and commuted to a major corporation daily. She usually left in the morning with just a cup of coffee or tea, grabbed a sandwich for lunch, and had a fast food dinner because she had no time to cook. Her husband usually brought in pizza, Kentucky Fried Chicken, or Burger King nightly and she cooked a little bit on the week-ends. She also noshed on the candy, chips, and ice cream that were in the house, and drank soda and alcohol occasionally.

Carol went to the gym at work sporadically where she did 20 minutes of cardio fitness. On week-ends Carol was usually busy with family obligations and chores and did not exercise.

In addition to help with weight loss, Carol wanted to improve her allergy symptoms, frequent sinus, and yeast infections. She did not like taking supplements and was just taking a one-a-day multiple.

Treatment

Carol's case was an example of someone headed straight towards Syndrome X. She had a family history of diabetes and heart disease and she was already obese. If she continued on her current path she most likely would be prone to disease in the near future.

It was challenging treating Carol, as well as many people like her, who work long hours and do not have a lot of time to prepare meals. In addition, Carol's husband consistently brought junk food into the house which was hard for her to resist.

Diet

During our first meeting I suggested that Carol make a few changes that she could control. I suggested she eat a balanced breakfast in the morning to boost her metabolism and help burn calories throughout the day. According to the March, 2004 *Tufts University Health and Nutrition Letter*, eating breakfast may curb overeating at night. In a study of 900 women and men, they found that eating a given number of calories earlier in the day proves more satiating than the same number of calories consumed later. In other words, by eating more at breakfast, the people in the study consumed fewer total calories for the day.

For breakfast, I recommended Carol pick something easy to grab that she could take to work such as a slice of whole grain toast with natural peanut butter, a hard boiled egg with a slice of high fiber bread, one cup of plain yogurt or cottage cheese with fresh fruit and ¼ cup almonds, or a protein drink with protein powder and organic skim or soy milk.

Since Carol consumed few vegetables throughout the day, I suggested she take advantage of her company salad bar at lunch and have a variety of vegetables or mixed greens with either chicken, turkey, beans, nuts, egg, or low-fat cheese on top. I recommended that Carol reduce her daily intake of starches. Lunch was a good meal to avoid them since there were a lot of other alternatives available.

For snacks, Carol kept trail mix and fruit at work so she wouldn't be tempted by the candy and chips that were easily accessible.

Carol's biggest challenge was what to eat for dinner during the week. She decided to buy a George Forman™ grill and cook chicken, fish, or low-fat meat, and sauté vegetables on the side using a non-stick pan. It only took 30 minutes to prepare a healthy dinner this way. She still consumed fast food with her family several times a week, but tried to choose the healthiest choices available.

Exercise

For exercise, Carol began walking at night several times a week and going to the gym at work more consistently. She was now going on the treadmill or stair machine for 30–40 minutes two to three times a week and working out with a personal trainer two times per week.

Supplements

Carol was resistant to taking a lot of vitamins, but I was able to recommend several that I thought were crucial to her weight loss success. She started taking L-Carnitine to burn fat more effectively and a formula called Glucose Regulation Complex* with chromium,* vanadium,* magnesium, alpha lipoic acid,* taurine* and zinc to help balance blood sugar and prevent sugar and carbohydrate cravings. I also recommended Vitamin C and garlic to help with Carol's allergies, sinus, and yeast infections. Garlic is a natural anti-viral, anti-bacterial, and anti-fungal herb.

Results

Over six months Carol lost 50 lbs. Her greatest success was in the first 3 months. Over the Christmas holidays she found it difficult to resist the abundance of candy and cookies available and gained back some weight. She got a fresh start in February, though, and lost an additional ten lbs.

One of Carol's greatest achievements was that she was slowly changing the eating habits of her family, who were all overweight. The nighttime walks became a family affair and everyone in the house ate more fruits, vegetables and less refined carbohydrates, sugar, and fat.

As Carol lost weight, ate healthier, and consistently exercised she felt better overall. She reported less moodiness and fatigue and some improvement in her allergy symptoms. Eating less sugar and wheat products as well as taking the supplements mentioned above, Carol greatly reduced her sinus and yeast infections.

Carol's Makeover: Before

Diet:	Ate on the run. Did not have breakfast. Ate fast food for dinner most nights. Noshed during the day on candy, chips and ice cream. Drank coffee, soda and alcohol regularly.
Weight/Cholesterol:	Carol's starting weight was 245, height 5'4, BMI =42. Cholesterol: Normal.
Triglycerides:	Triglycerides: Normal.
Supplements:	Carol was taking a one-a-day multiple vitamin to start.
Exercise:	Carol went to her company gym sporadically where she did some cardio-fitness. She had joint problems and found it hard to do too much.
Stress Mgt. & Self-Care:	Carol was under a huge amount of stress. She was the primary bread winner for her family and didn't really like her job. Her children were difficult and she had a strained relationship with her husband. She was anxious and cried easily. Carol was seeing a psychotherapist but was not doing any stress management or self-care techniques.

Carol's Makeover: After Total Wellness Program

Diet:	Balanced meal plan using 40/30/30 principles to keep her blood sugar steady and energy up. Carol now eats a healthy breakfast every day. Most carbohydrates consumed are low glycemic and high fiber. Portion sizes are moderate for grains and protein. Fruits, vegetables, whole grains, healthy fats and protein now make up the majority of Carol's diet. Carol still eats fast food, but limits herself to salads and grilled chicken. She snacks on nuts and fruit.

Weight/BMI:	Carol's weight was reduced to 187 after six months, BMI = 32.
Supplements:	Carol started on a multiple vitamin and a B-complex to help with her sugar cravings and stress. She added L-Carnitine and Vitamin C and garlic to help with her sinus and yeast infections.
Exercise:	Carol got serious about exercise and went to her company gym two to three times a week. She was able to do 20-30 minutes of cardio exercise and some strength and conditioning exercises. This improved her energy, stress level, and helped her to burn more calories and fat.
Stress Mgt. & Self-Care:	I encouraged Carol to keep a journal to record her feelings and daily frustrations, to address what she could change and accept what she could not. I also taught her some breathing techniques that she could use any where at any time to feel more relaxed. When I last saw her she was headed to a spa for a week-end by herself!

Summary

As illustrated in the above case histories, there are several keys to reversing the risk factors for Syndrome X and cardiovascular disease.

Step 1—Weight Management

Consume a diet low in saturated fat and refined carbohydrates. Increase fiber and water intake, and maintain a BMI of 25 or under. Weight management is so important for overall health and disease prevention, an entire chapter outlining my approach and a detailed food plan is provided in chapter 8. Studies show that as little as a 10% reduction in body weight, for instance a BMI from 31 to 28, will make a huge difference in the body's physiological response and ability to prevent disease. This is important not only for people at risk for Syndrome X, but for everyone.

Step 2—Exercise

A weekly exercise routine with at least 30 minutes of aerobic conditioning three times a week, and weight training two to three times a week works best for most people. It is really important to pick activities you enjoy such as walking, running, swimming, or bike riding. The key is consistency. Not only will this help with your cardiovascular fitness and assist in your weight loss or maintenance program, but it will also give you more energy, help you sleep better, and help you to manage stress more effectively. Always check with your doctor before starting a new exercise program.

Step 3—Supplements

There are many supplements that can be used to help prevent and reverse the diseases associated with Syndrome X. No one supplement program is right for everyone. We all have different bio-chemistries, genetic influences and life style factors that effect how many supplements we should take and in what doses. The following are general guidelines based on what has been effective for most of my patients. For more information, contact your doctor or nutritionist or check the resource section of this book. Do not go off any medication without first checking with your doctor.

Some of the supplements mentioned below can be found in foods. However, other than vitamin C, which is easiest to get from the diet, large quantities of the foods listed would have to be consumed, making it highly impractical to use just food as the source of these nutrients.

Key Heart Healthy Supplements

- **Coenzyme-Q10**—Provides cellular energy throughout the body and is a powerful antioxidant, particularly important in the treatment and prevention of cardiovascular disease. Studies have suggested that Co-Q10 can reduce the frequency of angina episodes, strengthen the heart muscle and increase the quality of life and survivability in those with congestive heart failure. Co-Q10 has also been shown to decrease blood pressure in patients with hypertension. Cholesterol lowering and statin drugs interfere with the production of Co-Q10. It is therefore especially important to take CoQ10 while using these drugs.

- **L-Carnitine**—Helps transport fatty acids into cells. By preventing fatty build-up, this amino acid aids in weight-loss, irregular heartbeats, heart arrhythmias, and angina. Carnitine can be manufactured in the body if sufficient amounts of lysine and iron are available. Lysine and iron are found mostly in meat, fish and poultry products. Vegetarians are the most at risk for carnitine deficiency.

- **B-Complex Vitamins**—Found mostly in meats, dairy, and whole grain products. Folate, B6 and B12 reduce homocysteine* levels, thought to increase the risk for heart disease.

- **Vitamin E** (mixed tocopherols is best)—Is a powerful anti-oxidant found in vegetable oils, wheat germ, nuts, and seeds. It keeps arteries clean and neutralizes free radicals. It is very difficult to get enough vitamin E from the diet alone. You would need to consume many cups of nuts or oil to get 400 IU's, which is the therapeutic dose most often recommended.

- **Magnesium**—Found mostly in vegetables, dairy and other animal products. It improves energy and oxygen production within the heart, inhibits blood clots, and improves heart rate and arrhythmias.

- **Vitamin C**—Found in citrus fruits, papaya, mango, and many vegetables. Can prevent oxidative damage to LDL cholesterol, and reduce its absorption into arterial walls.

Natural Cholesterol & Triglyceride Reducers

- **Soluble fiber**—Found in oat bran, barley, beans, and fruit. Lowers serum cholesterol by pulling it out of the body.

- **Flax or Fish Oil**—Reduces triglycerides and raises HDL, the good cholesterol that carries cholesterol and phospholipids from the cells back to the liver for recycling and disposal. Found to reduce the risk of death from coronary artery disease in some studies by as much as 50%.

- **Lecithin or phosphatidylcholine (PC)**—Found in soybean, liver, oatmeal, egg yolk, and some vegetables. Helps with cell membrane integrity and lowering triglycerides.

- **Soy Protein**—Inhibits absorption of cholesterol from the intestinal tract due to its ability to interfere with solubility of cholesterol, and inhibit bile acid re-absorption.

- **Niacin or Inositol Hexanicotinate** (non-flush kind)—Found in peanuts and brewers yeast, thought to lower cholesterol and triglycerides.

- **Gugulipid**—Improves LDL clearance from the body, inhibits LDL oxidation and adhesion.

- **Red Yeast Rice Extract**—Has been shown to promote healthy lipid levels by inhibiting a pathway for cholesterol production.

Supplements That Help With Pre-Diabetes and Diabetes

- **Fiber**—Keeps blood sugar stable and reduces the glycemic response.

- **Fish Oil**—Helps improve glucose and insulin metabolism.

- **Chromium**—Found in brewers yeast. Improves glucose tolerance in type-1 and type-2 diabetes by increasing sensitivity to insulin.

- **Alpha-lipoic acid**—Double blind studies have found that supplementing 600-1200 mg. of alpha lipoic acid per day improves insulin sensitivity and the symptoms of diabetic neuropathy.

- **Magnesium**—People with diabetes tend to have low magnesium levels. Magnesium supplementation has improved insulin production, particularly in elderly people with type-2 diabetes.

Stress Management

Like most disorders, heart disease, high blood pressure, and diabetes all have a stress component. In fact, it's hard to live in the world we do today without stress having some impact on our bodies. Many of my patients who are in their late 50's to late 70's tell me they have no stress because they are retired with their children no longer living at home. Yet, I see the stress of getting older, having sick friends, financial worries, or spousal conflict as very much a factor. Younger adults of course have family and career stress, and finding time to relax can be very difficult. Most of us have experienced daily stress for so long we no longer recognize it, but little by little it affects our health and should be looked at.

Stress to a large extent is biochemically mediated by our adrenal glands. These glands release cortisol and adrenaline in response to stress. In prehistoric days this was good—if we perceived a real threat, like being chased by a tiger, we would want lots of adrenaline to surge so we could run fast and escape or fight the animal. Nowadays, in our fast-paced stressful world the adrenal glands are so used to pumping out adrenaline and cortisol in response to daily life that we are in a constant state of fight or flight. This affects our health in many ways including our immune health, cardiovascular health, hormonal balance and all glands and tissues.

An interesting fact about stress and weight gain is that studies show that people who are in a constant "alarm state" store fat as a safety mechanism, particularly in their mid-section, which is most dangerous. This goes back to the prehistoric times when it wasn't always easy to find food. As with the hibernating animals, fat storage for later use became important.

That being said, incorporating some simple daily stress reduction exercises into your life like yoga, deep breathing, meditation or journal writing could be very helpful. I once had a biofeedback session at a health spa that I attended. While hooked up to a machine that monitored my stress level, I engaged in deep breathing exercises, meditation and writing for 15 minutes each. According to the results of the test, writing relaxed me the most. Since everybody is different, pick one or two activities that you find relaxing and do them daily to invoke a relaxation response. This response is necessary to lower cortisol levels and achieve better body balance. More examples will be discussed in chapter 11. The key is to slow down for at least 20 minutes every day and take time to relax and rejuvenate. It may be difficult to get started, but once you do the results will be significant and long-lasting.

3

Balance Hormones Naturally

Many of my patients have come in with hormonal imbalances over the years, and as I mentioned earlier, I personally have suffered with endometriosis and infertility.

The following are examples of types of conditions that could be caused or exacerbated by hormonal imbalance, either estrogen or progesterone that is too high or low, or another type of problem:

1. Endometriosis

2. Fibroids or cysts

3. Infertility

4. PCOD—Polycystic Ovarian Disease

5. PMS symptoms such as mood swings, depression, breast tenderness, headaches, cramping, and bloating

6. Perimenopausal symptoms such as anxiety, irritability, insomnia, frequent waking, and putting on weight more easily

7. Menopausal symptoms such as hot flashes, heavy bleeding, loss of libido, vaginal dryness, and memory loss

8. Frequent urinary tract infections, urinary incontinence, or interstitial cystitis* (a condition caused by chronic inflammation inside of the bladder)

9. All cancers influenced by excessive hormones including breast, ovarian, uterine, and endometrial cancer

Take this quiz to see if your diet and life style are most likely contributing to your hormonal concerns.

Hormone Balance Quiz

Each yes gets 1 point and no counts as 0.

1. Is your diet high in sugar and refined carbohydrates (white bread, white rice, white potato, pasta, cookies, cake, crackers, chips, pastries, high sugar cereals)? Count your servings per week—more than five gets a yes. A serving is ½ bagel, one slice of bread, ½ cup rice or pasta, 14 chips, ½ to one cup high sugar cereal, one baked potato, ten french fries, one piece of cake, one donut or pastry, one large or three small cookies.

2. Do you consume more than three glasses of alcohol a week?

3. Do you consume more than two caffeinated products a day? (Cup of coffee, tea, soda, or 1 oz. chocolate)

4. Do you eat more than two servings a week of meat (beef, pork) 3-4 oz., and full fat dairy products (hard cheese 1 oz., cream cheese 1 oz., whole milk 1 cup, 1 tbsp. butter) which are high in saturated fat?

5. Do you eat more than two servings a week of foods that are fried, processed, or cooked in hydrogenated or partially hydrogenated oils? Most cookies, crackers, and snack foods have hydrogenated or partially hydrogenated oils.

6. Are you currently on a low-fat diet? (Consuming less than 20 grams of fat a day).

7. Are you either overweight (BMI between 26-29), obese (BMI over 30) or underweight (BMI less than 20)?

8. Do you exercise too much (heavy exercise six-seven times a week) or not enough (less than three times a week)?

9. Have you been on birth control pills or have you ever taken hormones for infertility treatments for more than one year?

10. Do you take over-the-counter medications such as pain killers or antacids more than three times a week?

11. Do you eat more than five servings a week of foods sprayed with pesticides (non-organic fruits and vegetables) or antibiotics (chicken, beef, and pork fed antibiotics and growth hormones to increase their size)?

12. Have you had much exposure to toxic metals (lead, arsenic, cadmium, mercury, aluminum)? Traces of these toxic metals are found in our water and food supply. Cadmium is high in smokers or those exposed to second hand smoke. Aluminum is a preservative in baking powder, salad dressings, some commercial vitamins, and in most deodorants and personal care products. Mercury is found in large fish such as swordfish, shark and tuna. It is also in the preservative thimerisol, which has been used in many vaccinations and is currently in the flu shot.

Scoring and Rationale

1-3 Yes. You have good health habits, but your diet and life style may still be a contributing factor to your hormonal health problems now or in the future. Keep up the good work.

4-6 Yes. There is a good chance that your diet and life style may be contributing factors to your hormonal health problems now or in the future. Follow the dietary and life style recommendations in chapters 6-11 to improve your health.

Over 6 Yes. It is certain that there are some connections between your diet and life style and hormonal health problems. Follow the dietary and life style recommendations in chapters 6-11 to improve your health.

Rationale for Quiz

Questions 1-3. Poor diets with high sugar and white flour content and too much alcohol and caffeine are adrenal gland and hormonal depleters. This can cause fatigue, reduction of crucial nutrients that are necessary for hormone health, PMS, perimenopause, and menopause symptoms. There have also been several clinical studies linking alcohol and caffeine to an increased risk of infertility.

Questions 4-5. Eating too much meat and dairy, which are high in saturated fat, and hydrogenated or partially hydrogenated oils and fried foods can cause an essential fatty acid imbalance. Consuming a diet high in these fats offsets the balance of good fats in the body and has a negative effect on prostaglandins—the precursors for hormones.

Question 6. Low-fat diets can lead to not enough fat in the body; as more women try to lose weight and go on no-or low-fat diets they may not have enough cholesterol in the body to make healthy hormones. Having the right fats in the right amounts is crucial for hormonal balance.

Questions 7-8. Studies have shown that obese women have a greater risk of birth complications and children born with birth defects. They are also more likely to have trouble conceiving. In addition, too much or not enough exercise can be harmful. Women who run or do vigorous aerobic exercise consistently for long periods of time (such as marathon runners or tri-athletes) can adversely affect their sex drives and ovulation, creating an irregular cycle that is hard to get under control later when they are trying to get pregnant. Conversely, women who don't exercise at all or not enough will store more toxins in the body, not get enough blood flow to all key organs, and most likely will be above their ideal body weight, which in itself can cause hormonal imbalances.

Questions 9-10. Some conventional medications like birth control pills can have long-term effects on hormonal balance and fertility long after women stop taking them. Birth control pills and copper IUD's can offset the copper/zinc balance in the body causing copper toxicity* and depressed levels of zinc. Zinc is an important mineral for thyroid function and hormone production. Also, some antacids are high in aluminum and many of my patients take them frequently not realizing the high metal content. Instead of the body properly excreting aluminum, it can get stored and wreak havoc with the endocrine system.

Painkillers which can increase the risk of miscarriage, may also be potential problems. According to *The British Medical Journal,* August 16, 2003, pregnant women who use non-steroidal anti-inflammatory drugs (NSAIDS) and aspirin increase their risk of miscarriage by 80%. The risk is increased if the NSAID use took place around the time of conception or if the drugs were used for more than one week. Researchers suggest that the drugs suppress the production of prostaglandins, the fatty acid derivatives needed for successful implantation of an embryo into the womb. The drugs may lead to abnormal implantation and increase the chance the embryo will miscarry.

Another recent study is equally troubling. According to an article in the *Washington Post,* antibiotic usage may raise the risk for breast cancer. This study of more than 10,000 women in Washington State concluded that those who used the most antibiotics doubled their chances of developing breast cancer. Antibiotics affect bacteria in the digestive system in ways which interfere with how the body uses foods that protect against cancer. In addition, antibiotics may increase the risk of cancer by harming the immune system. The writers cautioned that more studies need to be conducted and that women should not stop taking life saving drugs when needed to treat infections.

Questions 11-12. Consuming foods high in outside estrogens can cause too much estrogen in the body. Properties from herbicides, PCB's, as well as from the hormones and antibiotics in our foods create strong xenoestrogens* that get stored and attached to the estrogen receptors in our bodies. The result: symptoms of excess estrogen such as endometriosis, fibroids, painful periods, and possibly breast cancer. In addition this can affect thyroid and pituitary function which are necessary for our reproduction organs to work properly.

Lead, arsenic, mercury, aluminum, cadmium, and other metals can interfere with ovulation and cause other hormonal imbalances. These things can come from smoking, household cleaners, paint fumes, gasoline, hair dyes, unclean water, amalgams, over the counter medications, personal care products, and foods such as fish from polluted waters. High consumption of fish contaminated with PCB's and mercury may reduce the ability of women to conceive and cause other health problems such as chronic fatigue, autoimmune diseases, and inflammation. If you suspect heavy metals in your body you may want to get a hair analysis or urine toxicity test. For more information, you can contact the labs in the resource section or check my website. There are now many products available that remove heavy metals from the body and help restore natural overall balance and hormonal health. Removal of heavy metals could be a complicated process, so please work with a qualified health care practitioner.

Complementary & Alternative Medicine for the Treatment of PMS, Painful Periods, Infertility and Menopause

Now that you have learned about many of the possible causes of poor hormonal health, let's discuss what can be done, and the latest clinical research.

In *The Reproductive Toxicology Journal, 2003,* doctors Adriane Fugh-Berman and Fredi Kronenberg review the randomized controlled trials available on common therapies for women's health issues like PMS, painful periods, and infertility. The following summarizes their published research. Keep in mind that the studies to date are limited. Since herbs, vitamins and other natural products cannot be patented, the funding for research is sparse.

PMS—33 randomized controlled trials were done using herbs, vitamins, minerals, manual therapies, diet, exercise, and mind-body approaches. The studies revealed the following:

- A multi-vitamin with B6 showed significant improvement in every category using London's 27 symptom menstrual questionnaire.

- Studies done on reducing dietary fat showed a significant effect on reducing water retention and the severity of pain associated with PMS.

- Increased aerobic exercise had a positive effect on improving PMS symptoms, but the same benefit was not seen in the strength/conditioning exercise group.

- Evidence suggests an overall symptom benefit for both calcium and magnesium, which are found to be lower in women with PMS.

- Chaste-tree berry, also named Vitex agnus-cactus, was shown in a study done with 178 women to help with symptoms of irritability, mood alteration, anger, headache, and breast fullness.

- A study of 30 women with severe PMS using evening primrose oil found that treatment reduced scores on a 19 point symptom scale significantly more than the control group.

- Manual therapies such as reflexology, massage, chiropractic adjustments, and mind-body treatment have also shown promising results.

Dysmenorrhea (Painful periods)—Thirteen small studies were noted in the article. Of those, the most promising data was on fish oils

(EPA and DHA), exercise, a low-fat/vegetarian diet, vitamin E, and acupuncture.

Infertility—Of the limited studies done, the one cited in the above mentioned article was a randomized double-blind placebo-controlled trial of 52 women with luteal phase defect* associated with high pro-lactin* levels. Vitex extract (20 mg./day) reduced prolactin levels, and normalized luteal phase length and progesterone levels. In a different article, *Journal of Reproductive Medicine,* April, 2004, positive findings were illustrated in a double-blind, placebo controlled study using a fer-tility blend of vitex, green tea extracts, L-arginine, and vitamins and minerals. In this study 30 women aged 24-46 who were unable to con-ceive for six-36 months showed increases in mean midluteal phase progesterone levels and the average number of days in the cycle. After five months, five out of the 15 women in the supplement group were pregnant (33%) and none of the 15 women in the placebo group.

Menopause—Many alternative therapies have been studied for menopause. Those with the most positive clinical data are black cohosh, red clover, soy and flax oil.

- One study published in *Obstetrics Gynecology,* 2002 found flax-seed supplementation about as effective in controlling a variety of menopausal symptoms as standard doses of hormone replace-ment therapy. Flaxseeds may also have additional cardiovascular benefits and may be protective against breast cancer.

- In *The Annals of Internal Medicine,* November, 2002, several complementary treatments for menopause were looked at. Soy remains controversial, but the referenced studies have shown it to reduce hot flashes significantly. Caution should be used espe-cially for women with a prior history of cancer.

- Several controlled trials support the use of black cohosh for menopausal symptoms. It is recommended for short term use only until more information is assessed regarding possible endometrial stimulation or estrogenic effect on breast tissue. According to expert Dr. Adriane Fugh-Berman, women using this herb should be followed with vaginal ultrasound and possible endometrial biopsy to minimize possible risks.

- Red clover has been minimally studied; two randomly controlled trials show that it is beneficial for hot flashes.

Now let's put this information to practical use by illustrating four makeover examples using many of the recommendations studied.

Angela's Health Makeover: Infertility & PMS

Background

Angela came to see me after reading an article I wrote about natural approaches to infertility. She was 39 at the time and had recently completed several cycles of hormones with inseminations and finally a failed IVF (in vitro fertilization) that left her emotionally and physically drained. She also had severe PMS symptoms, specifically anxiety and depression, about two weeks before her period. According to Angela, she felt like a different person during that time with doubts about her work and productivity. Her doctor was recommending an anti-depressant to get her through this difficult time, but she really wanted to go the natural route first. In addition, she always had a bad reaction to sugary and fatty foods, getting cramping and diarrhea. In her work she traveled a lot and didn't eat or sleep well while away. She also had been exposed to mercury several years prior and had a mouth full of mercury amalgams.

Treatment

At the first meeting we worked on Angela's diet, which was good when she wasn't traveling. I recommended a plan of three balanced meals and two snacks to keep her blood sugar and energy level steady throughout the day, as well as more quality protein, vegetables, nuts and flax oil. Since she had been trying to get pregnant, sugar and alcohol were already reduced in her diet. Previously Angela was taking a multi-vitamin and B-complex. I suggested she add: vitamin E, which protects hormones and reproductive organs from free-radical damage, vitamin C, which has been shown to prevent age-related reduction in ovulation and help prevent miscarriage, gamma linoleic acid (GLA), an essential fatty acid, which helps with all aspects of female reproductive health, especially cramping, irritability, headaches and water retention, and finally a probiotic* supplement to help with her cramping and diarrhea. We also did a hair analysis to make sure the earlier toxic metal exposure was no longer a problem.

When Angela came back to see me in three weeks her energy and sleep were much improved and her cycle seemed better. We went over her hair analysis, which revealed a copper/zinc imbalance, low levels of most minerals across the board, low sodium and potassium which usually indicates adrenal exhaustion, and finally an elevated aluminum level. The first problem to tackle was the copper/zinc imbalance. Excessive copper in the tissues is commonly associated with menstrual problems as copper interferes with normal thyroid function, essential for normal periods. In addition, available copper is necessary for ovulation and fertilization and one of the consequences of copper imbalance is changes in acidity and dryness of the vaginal mucosa, which impairs sperm motility. High copper levels are also implicated with PMS symptoms. Infertility may be triggered by a relative deficiency of progesterone in relation to estrogen. Estrogen levels rise as copper rises, thus Angela's high copper levels were one contributing factor bringing up her estrogen levels and resultant relative progesterone deficiency.

There was now a lot more information to work with for her treatment. The best way to balance out copper is to add zinc. I recommended an additional zinc supplement as well as a stress formula to help with the adrenal burnout symptoms.

Results

On her return visit one month later, Angela reported feeling much better. The PMS symptoms were completely gone. She also had much better digestion and was now able to tolerate the occasional dessert without ramifications.

Angela felt she no longer needed treatment and was hoping to conceive naturally since she felt so much better and was certain that her body was back in balance. Had she continued to see me the next step was to do a saliva hormone profile using 11 samples over 28 days, to see what her actual levels of estrogen, progesterone, and testosterone were. While most doctors use blood tests to check hormone levels, the saliva test is less expensive, more convenient as it is done at home, and more comprehensive since it tracks the hormones throughout the entire cycle instead of just one day. If you would like more information about this type of test, check the resource section of the book.

Angela's Makeover: Before

Problem: PMS, infertility, digestion	Anxiety, depression two weeks before period. Several failed IUI's and one IVF. Could not eat sugary or fatty foods without a gastrointestinal episode.
Diet:	High carbohydrate to protein ratio. Meals were not balanced, which resulted in fatigue and cravings for sugary foods, especially during her period.
Supplements:	Multi-vitamin and B complex.
Exercise:	Exercised inconsistently.
Stress Mgt. & Self-Care:	Had a great deal of stress with work and infertility treatments. Had no formal program to de-compress her emotions.

Angela's Makeover: After Total Wellness Program

Problem: PMS, infertility, digestion	Cycle improved. Much less anxiety and depression before her period. When we last spoke Angela was feeling so much better she was trying to get pregnant naturally. She was also able to eat the occasional high fat foods without any problems.
Diet:	Recommended a balanced plan with three meals and two snacks. Added more protein, vegetables, nuts, and flax oil to Angela's diet.
Supplements:	Added vitamin E, C, GLA, probiotics, and an adrenal support/ stress formula on a short term basis.
Exercise:	Angela began going to the gym three times a week and walking on the week-ends.
Stress Mgt. & Self-Care:	I encouraged Angela to take a yoga class and write in a journal nightly before bed to release any stress or pent up anxiety she was having.

Maria's Health Makeover: Interstitial Cystitis & Perimenopause

Background

Maria was referred to me by her urologist over four years ago. She had just been diagnosed with interstitial cystitis (IC), a chronic bladder disease caused by inflammation in the bladder walls that causes urinary frequency, burning, pelvic heaviness or pain, and in some cases can be so severe that the urge to urinate occurs every 30-60 minutes. That's how severe Maria's symptoms were when she first came to see me. She was 45 at the time, which put her into the age group when many women start to experience hormonal changes. In addition to the bladder problem she was experiencing fatigue, food allergies, night sweats, sinus problems, mood swings, and depression. She had been on Prozac for her depression and was in tears during our meeting wondering how she was going to cope with this new illness.

Treatment

Since I have worked with many IC patients over the years, I was able to give Maria reassurance that by changing her diet and adding some key anti-inflammatory supplements, she would feel better soon. As an Italian, Maria consumed a lot of red sauces and tomatoes, two of the worst foods for IC, due to high acid content. I also recommended that she remove other acidic foods like coffee, alcohol, vinegar, citrus fruits, and other foods that are irritants like cheese, dried fruit, avocado, nuts, and chocolate from her diet. I explained to Maria that these foods needed to be eliminated for a short time (usually one-three months) to allow the inflammation in her bladder to be repaired. When she was feeling better, foods could be added back in moderation without any problem.

It was also important for Maria to improve her sleep so she could better handle her anxiety and stress, which were exacerbating the IC symptoms. I recommended acupuncture treatments and relaxation exercises as an adjunct to the nutritional program.

The supplements that were recommended for Maria were a multi-vitamin/mineral complex for overall balance, a non-acidic vitamin C for her sinus problems, vitamin E for night sweats and allergies, fish oil for inflammation and depression, calcium/magnesium for anxiety and relaxing the bladder muscles, and a probiotic supplement to make sure there wasn't extra bacteria or yeast that were making her symptoms worse. I recommended the following tests for Maria: a food sensitivity panel, since many people with IC have food intolerances; a hormone saliva profile since I suspected that her hormones were playing a major role in the anxiety/depression; and blood work to rule out anemia and thyroid problems.

Results

On her follow-up visit, Maria reported that she thought the diet would be much harder than it was. She was feeling a lot better with more energy, longer sleep without night sweats, and less frequency and burning when she urinated. The blood work showed slight anemia and no thyroid problems. The food sensitivity test showed problems with cow's milk, aspartame, wheat, garlic, banana, lentils, cashews, and certain vegetables. Her hormone test revealed estrogen at the low end of normal with no mid-cycle surge, an elevated progesterone level, and normal testosterone levels.

The next phase of Maria's program was to customize her diet based on the food test for a period of 90 days so that the sensitive foods could be removed from her system, allowing her body to heal. Because of the low iron levels, I recommended that Maria add more meat, fish, and poultry to her meal plan since these are the best sources of natural iron. For her low estrogen levels, I suggested she add more plant estrogens to her diet like soy and flax, and try using chasteberry extract, an adaptive herb* that helps with hormone balance.

Summary

Over a period of several years I have seen Maria on and off. For the most part she is managing her IC and emotional symptoms well. She occasionally calls for a visit when she goes off of her diet and supplements and starts experiencing a flare-up of symptoms. This is common for patients with IC. When they closely follow the diet and take their supplements regularly most of them feel normal again in a matter of a few months. Many are then able to tolerate a little citrus fruit or a glass of wine without consequence. It is having the motivation to make the change in the first place that is the most difficult. As Maria is nearing 50 she has had few menopausal symptoms other than some anxiety and depression once in a while which she feels she can tolerate. Overall, her diet, supplements and life style changes have served her well and she is maintaining good health and balance. When we last spoke, Maria had gone back to work full-time and was energetic and able to handle her daily stress better. She is currently working with her doctor to wean herself off of Prozac.

Maria's Makeover: Before

Problem: Interstitial cystitis (IC), fatigue, food allergies, perimenopause symptoms.	Maria had pain and urinary frequency. She was anxious, with night sweats, sinus problems, fatigue, mood swings, and some depression. She was also sleep deprived and not sure what foods were safe for her newly diagnosed medical condition.
Diet:	She consumed a lot of red sauces and tomatoes, highly acidic foods which were inflaming her bladder condition. She also drank a lot of coffee and consumed a fair amount of sugar and refined grains.
Supplements:	Centrum multi and vitamin C.
Exercise:	Was not able to exercise after her IC diagnosis.
Stress Mgt. & Self-Care:	Had a great deal of stress dealing with this new illness as well as some personal stuff going on with her extended family. She had a lot of support from her husband but no formal program for stress management.

Maria's Makeover: After Total Wellness Program

Problem: IC, perimenopause symptoms, food sensitivities & fatigue	Maria found that the IC diet was easier to follow than she anticipated so much of her anxiety improved. She was sleeping through the nights with minimal night sweats and only getting up once to urinate. Her energy and overall vitality improved substantially.
Diet:	Recommended a balanced plan with three meals and two snacks. Per her food challenge test, Maria removed the foods that she was sensitive to as well as acidic and other foods that cause a problem for IC.
Supplements:	Switched her multi to an all natural one with no artificial colors or preservatives. Added vitamin E, non-acidic vitamin C, EPA/DHA, GLA, and B-complex to help with Maria's ongoing stress and anxiety.

Exercise:	Maria began running three times a week and walking on the weekends.
Stress Mgt. & Self-Care:	Maria started acupuncture, which relaxed her and helped with the IC symptoms. She also prayed and spent quality time with her husband and children.

Michelle's Health Makeover: Infertility, Perimenopause & Weight Management

Background

Michelle came to see me after reading an article I wrote about infertility in a journal. The following are excerpts from her letter which accompanied the questionnaire that I ask all patients to fill out with information about their background and history before our first meeting:

"My husband and I have been trying to get pregnant for many years after moving back from France several years ago. We have worked with three fertility specialists for over three years and then after just beginning an IVF program, decided to call it quits and adopt. The doctors only gave us a small chance of success through IVF as my FSH levels are consistently high, although they cannot find anything wrong. We are happy about the decision to adopt and are moving on but I feel that my weight and my nutrition are still large issues. When I read your article it spoke to me on two levels 1) taking charge of my own health and well being and 2) should we be lucky, getting pregnant. I would like to work with you with both goals in mind, however, should getting pregnant not be in the cards, I will be equally happy just taking care of myself."

Michelle was an ideal patient because she embodied the total wellness concepts and couldn't wait to take charge of her health and put them into practice. During our initial interview she revealed that she wanted to improve her energy level and handle stress better as well as the goals mentioned in the letter. Michelle was 38 and weighed close to 200 lbs on a 5'10" frame. She complained that she looked and felt much older than she actually was and tied her recent weight gain to leaving France and eating the standard American diet with reduced exercise. She also felt that the stress of the infertility treatments and leaving a job she really liked in France were driving her to eat. This was an example where stress was not only affecting Michele's weight but her whole bio-chemistry.

Treatment

As usual, we started by looking at Michelle's diet. Her breakfast started with two pieces of plain toast or a fruit and yogurt smoothie. For lunch she had either a ham or a turkey sandwich, or leftover pasta. If nothing was around she would have toast again for lunch. For dinner she had pasta with or without meat, chicken with rice and vegetables, or soup with bread. Her snacks were apple sauce, yogurt, or when there was nothing in the house, you guessed it, toast. Although she didn't keep a lot of junk food in the house, several times a week her husband would bring home cookies and they would eat them until they were finished. She had already cut out caffeine and alcohol as part of her program to try to get pregnant.

It was clear that Michelle's diet contained too many carbohydrates, contributing to her fatigue and weight gain, and not enough protein and healthy fats to keep her energy up, cravings down, and hormones stable. I recommended that Michelle change her diet to incorporate protein with each meal and two healthy snacks to keep her blood sugar balanced and energy steady. By adding protein powder and flax seeds to her fruit and yogurt smoothie, or natural peanut or almond butter to her toast there was a big improvement to her breakfast, giving her more energy and filling her up. Whereas carbohydrates alone create a quick surge in energy and then a quick drop, when eaten with protein or fat the release of energy is more gradual and sustained and hunger delayed. We added some other choices for breakfast as well such as oatmeal with a scoop of protein powder, and some almonds, or one or two eggs with one slice of whole grain toast or a fruit.

For lunch I suggested salads with protein (chicken, turkey, beans, or low-fat cheese) and for dinner 4 oz. of lean meat, fish, or poultry with a vegetable, and salad with small starch portion. Snacks were ¼ cup nuts with fruit, one oz. low-fat cheese or turkey rolled up with mustard, or half of a protein bar. They are usually around 200 calories so you have to be careful when using them as a snack. It is also important to watch the amount of corn syrup and hydrogenated oils that are prevalent in many energy bars. I recommended that Michelle also increase her water intake to 64 oz a day and supplement with herbal tea such as red raspberry, which is thought to have a positive hormonal effect.

Michelle decided to walk five days a week at a town park that was fairly hilly and would provide good aerobic conditioning. She was used to doing a lot of walking in France, and this would provide a good way for her to enjoy the outdoors again. I also recommended yoga for relaxation, stretching and toning, and gave her a meditation tape.

For testing we started with a mineral analysis/toxic metal screening to see if there were any specific nutrient imbalances that could be affecting her energy or hormone levels. The results of this test would show nutrient deficiencies, copper/zinc imbalance, heavy metals, and how her adrenal and thyroid glands were functioning.

The supplement that Michelle decided to start with were a liver cleanser with milk thistle, dandelion, artichoke, and reishi mushroom. I find that cleansing the liver is very important to help with hormone balance issues. I also recommended an all natural multi-vitamin and mineral supplement, B-complex for stress and energy, gamma linoleic acid (GLA), an essential fatty acid for hormone balance and vitamins C, E, and zinc for hormone regulation and immune system enhancement.

When Michelle returned three weeks later she had lost a few lbs and was starting to feel better. Her mineral/toxic metal test revealed low electrolytes (calcium, magnesium, sodium and potassium), a high copper/zinc ratio, and low levels of chromium and zinc which are needed for blood sugar balance. Toxic metals did not seem to be an issue at the time of the test.

We decided to work on improving Michelle's sodium and potassium levels helping her adrenal glands function better, improving fatigue, and removing excess tissue copper from organ storage. Excess copper could slow the metabolism, impact the thyroid gland, and affect hormone balance. I recommended adding an electrolyte drink without sugar to improve the four low electrolytes, a glandular extract to improve adrenal function, and the minerals zinc and chromium to help with blood sugar balance and fat, protein, and carbohydrate metabolism regulation. These things are used temporarily as the levels even out and should be stopped when symptoms improve or repeat testing shows they are no longer needed.

Results

I continued to see Michelle every one to three months over two years. She lost 40 lbs., her FSH (follicle stimulating hormone, one benchmark used by reproductive endocrinologists to see how fertile a woman is) dropped to normal levels. In addition, Michelle reported an improved energy and stress level, and she looked and felt years younger. On our last visit, Michelle gave me the news that she had just adopted a baby girl. The following are excerpts from a parting letter she wrote me:

"I have lost weight and feel so much better. I am exercising and getting myself back in shape. I went hiking with my dad and climbed a nearby mountain that I have climbed before, but this time instead of huffing and puffing the entire way with frequent rest stops, I raced up. It felt great to get the old me back again! Also, my husband thinks I look ten years younger. My family, particularly my mom, who used to worry about me, thinks I look great. Most importantly, I feel great, like the old me!"

Michelle's Makeover: Before

Problem: Infertility, weight issues, fatigue, stress management	Michelle had been to many infertility specialists and had three failed attempts at getting pregnant. She was anxious to improve her overall health and well being and to lose some weight.
Diet:	She consumed a diet high in carbohydrates, particularly white bread and pasta. She had a weakness for ice cream and cookies and since her husband traveled a lot didn't bother to cook regular healthy meals for herself.
Supplements:	Prenatal vitamin.
Exercise:	Used to exercise a lot but was too fatigued to exercise lately.
Stress Mgt. & Self-Care:	Michelle did a lot of volunteer work and was also trying to find a paying job. Most of her stress was from moving and leaving a job that she really liked because of her husband's career. She also felt great stress from not being able to have a child. She was currently doing a yoga program and found it was helping somewhat with her stress and anxiety levels.

Michelle's Makeover: After Total Wellness Program

Problem: Infertility, weight gain, fatigue, stress management	Michelle decided to stop her infertility treatments and to adopt a baby. This gave her much happiness and relieved a lot of her stress related symptoms. After changing her diet and supplement program and adding a significant amount of exercise, Michelle lost 40 lbs. and felt so much better in terms of her energy and overall wellness.
Diet:	Recommended a balanced plan with three meals and two snacks. Adding more protein and healthy fats and reducing carbohydrates worked well for Michelle. It gave her a boost in energy and reduced her cravings for sweets. Ice cream, cookies, bread, and pasta became occasional treats instead of the bulk of her diet.
Supplements:	Started Michelle on a cleansing program which included a product with milk thistle, dandelion, artichoke, and reishi mushroom. Switched her prenatal to an all natural one with no artificial colors or preservatives and more minerals than what is normally in a prenatal. Added vitamin E, vitamin C, EPA/DHA, GLA, and B-complex to help with Michelle's fatigue and stress.
Exercise:	Michelle began swimming and walking her dogs in a hilly park four-five times a week. This improved her energy, helped her to lose weight, and reduced her stress.
Stress Mgt. & Self-Care:	Michelle continued her yoga program, and added several meditation and visualization exercises.

Lisa's Health Makeover: Infertility, Miscarriage, Insomnia, & Poor Hair Growth

Background

Lisa came to see me after she had four failed attempts at artificial insemination and two attempts at in vitro fertilization that resulted in pregnancy and miscarriage. She was 43 years old, tall and thin. In addition to wanting to achieve a full term pregnancy, Lisa was having sleep problems and was therefore always tired.

Her diet lacked sufficient protein, especially for breakfast, as well as fruits, vegetables, and essential fatty acids. She had sweets cravings after lunch and dinner and usually ate ice cream and chocolate during the day to "feel better."

Treatment

I recommended Lisa improve her energy by eating three balanced meals and two snacks with protein in each. This would help with her sugar cravings by keeping her blood sugar stable. I also suggested she add foods high in essential fatty acids to her diet such as flax meal or oil and wild salmon to help stabilize hormone levels.

The supplements I recommended were a natural multi-vitamin and mineral complex, B Complex to help with stress, energy, and sugar cravings, GLA for hormone balance, vitamins C and E, which have been found to be protective against miscarriage, and calcium and magnesium, calming nutrients to help with sleep and stress.

Hormone saliva and mineral/toxic metal tests were ordered to get a better understanding of why Lisa couldn't sleep and wasn't able to sustain a pregnancy.

Lisa's mineral/toxic metal test revealed small levels of mercury and aluminum, and poor adrenal and thyroid function, indicated by low sodium and potassium levels. Adrenal insufficiency is a common cause of poor hair growth. Lisa also had a high calcium to magnesium ratio which was causing an insulin imbalance resulting in an inability to properly metabolize sugar and carbohydrates as well as sugar cravings. In addition, Lisa's chromium and manganese levels were low which was also indicative of problems regulating blood sugar.

According to her hormone test, Lisa had a normal ovulation cycle, indicated by an adequate estradiol peak followed by a rise of progesterone in the peak range. Her testosterone and estradiol levels were also in the normal range during the whole month. She had elevated progesterone in the early part of her cycle, which can be due to adrenal dysfunction or heavy metals (consistent with other test), and a luteal phase defect. This means inadequate amounts of progesterone available mid cycle to sustain a pregnancy. This can be due to adrenal insufficiency* and free-radical damage.* As a result of the tests, I recommended Lisa add an adrenal complex to her program and a product to help regulate blood sugar. I also suggested extra vitamin C, and added selenium, garlic, and glutathione* to help remove the toxic metals from her system.

Results

Over the next several months Lisa followed the dietary recommendations and reduced her sugar intake except for an occasional cookie. She no longer had sweet cravings, was sleeping better, with improved energy and nicer quality skin and hair. Her periods were also better with less cramping and clotting. Lisa's doctors were pleased that her FSH levels dropped, and she would be a candidate to do another IVF cycle.

Although drug therapy was always difficult in the past, this time Lisa reported fewer mood swings and less fatigue while taking her hormone stimulating drugs. She got pregnant and delivered a health baby boy with little trouble.

Lisa's Makeover: Before

Problem: Infertility, miscarriage, insomnia, poor hair growth	Lisa had conceived several times, but her pregnancies always ended in miscarriage. She was stressed, had trouble sleeping, and noticed that her hair was easily falling out.
Diet:	Lisa consumed an average diet that lacked sufficient protein and essential fatty acids. She often craved sweets and ate chocolate and ice cream to boost energy in the afternoon.
Supplements:	Prenatal vitamin.
Exercise:	Lisa walked three-four times a week.
Stress Mgt. & Self-Care:	Lisa had a high degree of stress from the frequent miscarriages. She also had a fair amount of stress from her work and family. She was not currently doing anything proactive to relieve her stress.

Lisa's Makeover: After Total Wellness Program

Problem: Infertility, miscarriage, hair loss, insomnia	After several tests we found Lisa to have certain hormone and mineral imbalances that were contributing to her symptoms. She also had some toxic metals. After changing her diet and supplement program and learning to relax more, Lisa got pregnant and was able to sustain the pregnancy. She was also sleeping better, had more energy, and improved hair growth.
Diet:	Recommended a balanced plan with three meals and two snacks. Adding more protein and healthy fats and reducing carbohydrates worked well for Lisa. It gave her a boost in energy and reduced her cravings for sweets. Ice cream and chocolate became occasional treats and were no longer needed to boost her energy in the afternoon.
Supplements:	Lisa started on a better health program with a good multi vitamin, vitamins E,C, EPA/DHA, GLA, and B-complex. Once we got Lisa's test results, we added several supplements to help reduce the toxic metals in her system and improve her hormone balance.

Exercise:	Lisa continued walking and added some light weight training. This improved her energy and stress level.
Stress Mgt. & Self-Care:	I recommended that Lisa join a support group for women who have had multiple miscarriages. This seemed to help her cope better. I also taught her some meditation and relaxation exercises and how to visualize her health improved.

Summary

The following is a summary of what I have found to work with almost all of my patients over the years with just about any problem relating to hormone balance. Many have gotten pregnant who thought they never would, with or without simultaneous infertility treatments. In addition, debilitating PMS and perimenopausal symptoms have been resolved, and for those who have started the program early enough, a smooth transition into menopause.

- Life Style factors:

  1. Quit Smoking.

  2. Get chemicals out of your house and body including household cleaners, and pesticides, hormones, additives, and preservatives from foods. Remove toxic metals like lead, mercury, and aluminum from your body.

  3. Reduce or eliminate over-the-counter drugs.

- Diet:

  4. Reduce consumption of fish contaminated with PCB's and mercury.

  5. Eat for hormone balance choosing foods high in phytoestrogens and essential fatty acids. Diet should be balanced consisting of mostly quality protein, steamed vegetables, fresh fruit, whole grains, nuts, beans, and seeds.

6. Drink 64 ounces of water a day to help with natural detoxification. Sodas contain phosphorus which depletes calcium and other minerals from your bones and should be eliminated. Many people who think they are hungry or tired are really dehydrated so drink water religiously to help with fatigue and weight balance.

7. Reduce or eliminate caffeine, alcohol and white sugar.

8. Eliminate hydrogenated or partially hydrogenated oils, fried and processed foods, and artificial sweeteners, dyes, and colors.

9. Maintain an ideal body weight, not too thin and not too heavy. Optimal weight is a body mass index of 20-25.

- Exercise:

10. Exercise at least 30-45 minutes, three times a week. Some activity daily is ideal.

- Supplements:

11. Take some vitamins/minerals. The following are the basic vitamins that I recommend for hormonal health. The regimen is best individualized based on the background, history and presenting symptoms:

  - Multi-vitamin/mineral complex with enough zinc, selenium, and chromium which tends to be low for many individuals. I recommend it with iron for those still menstruating and without iron after menopause.

  - B-Complex—make sure there is enough B6 which helps with water retention and other PMS symptoms

  - Vitamin C

  - Vitamin E

  - Calcium/Magnesium with vitamin D

  - EPA/DHA or flax oil

- GLA

12. I recommend using the following herbs for certain problems:

- Red raspberry—a natural female tonic and fertility booster

- Chasteberry Extract or Vitex*—thought to help regulate menstrual cycles, the ovary's production of estrogen and progesterone, and help with elevated levels of prolactin.*

- Dong quai—An herb that may act as a female tonic to balance hormones and uterine muscles. Helps to regulate menstrual cycles and ease cramps.

- Black cohosh—An herb which can have an estrogen-like action and help with menstrual symptoms related to low estrogen production.

In addition to these herbs and supplements, some of my patients have digestive issues, liver problems, or heavy metals which need to be removed before the above program is effective. That is why it is important to work with a qualified health care practitioner and get testing done if needed to ensure that you are off to the right start.

- Stress Management and Self-Care:

13. Find joy, peace and laughter every day in your current life. Through hobbies, pets, supportive friends, relatives, and spouses go to your bliss station every day. Make sure that your daily life includes activities that are fun and enjoyable—not just work and chores.

14. Find stress reducers that you like such as yoga, meditation, tai chi, taking warm baths, walks in the woods, journal writing, or getting weekly massages and do them consistently, for at least

20 minutes a day. Chapter 11 is devoted to stress management tips.

4

Improve Digestive Health

Over the years, I have seen many patients with digestive health issues. Often the patient comes to me for another problem like skin eruptions or chronic fatigue and during the detailed patient interview, digestive issues are uncovered that the patient has lived with for so long, he or she considers them normal. Without digestive health there cannot be a healthy immune system or overall total wellness. Without healthy digestion nutrients needed to feed all of the cells in the body will not be properly absorbed and utilized. When people who are sick and also have digestive problems take the path of consuming a lot of vitamins, they will probably be wasting their money since most of these nutrients will never get into the blood stream. If a patient comes to see me with a host of problems and one of them has to do with digestion, I always recommend that we start there first.

The most common digestive complaints are:

- Constipation
- Diarrhea
- Yeast overgrowth/Candida*
- Irritable bowel syndrome*
- Gastric reflux*
- Crohn's* or colitis*
- Food allergies/sensitivities

There is a formula that many natural health care practitioners use when there is a problem in the digestive tract. It is called the 4 R's program: remove, replace, re-introduce and repair. That simply means remove the things that are causing the problem such as bacteria, parasites, candida or yeast overgrowth, and foods that one is sensitive or reactive to. Replace the diet with healthy food, fiber, and pure water for regular elimination. Re-introduce the gut with probiotics to put healthy micro flora* into the system, and digestive enzymes if needed to assist with the breakdown of protein, fats, and carbohydrates in the diet. Lastly, repair the gut lining so food and germs do not get through to the blood stream and cause a bad reaction. This is called "leaky gut syndrome" and is thought to cause all kinds of problems from food allergies to irritable bowel syndrome, and colitis. It is frequently seen with high dose antibiotic usage. The antibiotics essentially cause cells protecting the gut to die. The intestinal barrier pulls apart and causes things foreign to the blood to leak through.

I have seen this formula work over and over again for many years, hearing responses from patients like "I feel like I have someone else's stomach," or "In my whole life I never thought I would get rid of my chronic gas and bloating." It may take two or three months to get this kind of result, but for the patients who follow the recommendations, the result that they want is usually attainable.

This process should not be understated. According to Doctor Nigel Plummer who has been studying the role of micro flora in the digestive tract for years, normal micro flora:

- Stimulates maturation and balancing of the immune system at birth and then stimulates and primes the immune system throughout life. In other words, if we don't acquire enough normal micro flora at birth and never correct the problem, we will have a compromised immune system for life. This important point will be elaborated on in the next chapter on children's health.

- Provides protection against infection. For instance, if our normal beneficial flora is attached to intestinal epithelial tissue, then bad bacteria, yeast and parasites cannot attach.

- Synthesizes vitamins, particularly the B vitamins: B12, Folic Acid, Biotin, Riboflavin, and vitamin K. These important vitamins are needed for many metabolic functions in the body.

- Synthesizes short chain fatty acids (SCFA'S). It is estimated that five-ten % of the total body energy is from SCFA'S. Without them, there is a decrease in the integrity of the mucosal lining protecting the gut and a greater chance of the "leaky gut syndrome" that was discussed earlier to occur.

- Detoxifies toxins such as heavy metals by binding to them and facilitating excretion from the body.

- Releases quercetin* from fruit and transforms plant compounds releasing phytoestrogens (iso-flavones).* Quercetin and rutin have been shown to be powerful anti-mutagens. Iso-flavones have been shown to be protective against colon and breast cancer.

If there is one digestive supplement that everyone with gastrointestinal problems can benefit from it is probiotics, or beneficial flora. The most popular strains are lactobacillus acidophilus and bifido bacteria.

More on this and other beneficial supplements for digestive health will be discussed in the following makeover examples.

Lee's Health Makeover—Irritable Bowel, Candida, Poor Diet

Background

Lee was visiting from down south when she came to my office. She was 56 at the time, about 25 lbs. overweight and complaining of colitis with bad gas, bowel movement urgency, and loose stools to the point where she was afraid to do much traveling, which she had really enjoyed in the past. In addition to seeing me, she went to a top gastro-enterologist in New York City. She was otherwise in excellent health except for some arthritis that bothered her mostly at night.

The doctor gave Lee a colonoscopy which was basically normal, diagnosed her with irritable bowel, and sent her on her way. Her diet was high in sugar and fat, and low in vegetables, protein, and fiber.

Treatment

I recommended reducing Lee's consumption of meat and dairy, which are pro-inflammatory (contributing to her gut inflammation and arthritis), and eliminating alcohol, wheat and sugar, which tend to be gut irritants, for four weeks.

The meal plan that I provided was high in fiber consisting of whole grains (other than wheat), legumes, vegetables, fruits, nuts and seeds as well as quality protein, with lots of purified water to help push the fiber through her digestive tract. Wheat was withdrawn initially because it can cause irritation to the gastrointestinal system and is the grain that many people are most sensitive to. It might seem odd to the reader to recommend fiber when there are loose stools, but sometimes this is the result of not enough bulk to create a healthy bowel movement. In addition, Lee started on an acidophilus/bifidobacteria supplement to build healthy gut flora and reduce bacterial overgrowth, and pepper-mint-ginger tablets to help with the daily symptoms of gas and bloat-ing. I asked her to record what she ate and how she was feeling and gave her a stool collection kit.

The specialty lab that I use looks for things like how much good bacteria are available, whether proper digestion and absorption are tak-ing place based on certain markers, and if any bad bacteria, pathologi-cal yeast, or parasites are causing a problem. Information about this lab is also in the resource section or on my website.

When Lee and I did a phone follow-up several weeks later she informed me that her gas and bloating were much improved and her bowel urgency was somewhat better although she still had loose stools.

According to the test results, Lee had elevated levels of cholesterol in her stool which may reflect fat malabsorption, too much dietary cholesterol, fiber insufficiency, or intestinal inflammation. With the changes she already made in her diet, I thought these problems would resolve without further treatment. She had decreased levels of short-chain fatty acids, which are crucial for the health of the intestine and serve as fuel for the cells and the rest of the body. Insufficient amounts may reflect not enough healthy flora, a diet low in fiber, or not enough butyrate which provides energy for colon cells. Meat and vegetable fibers were seen in the stool, direct indicators of malabsorption due to hydrochloric acid or pepsin insufficiency (digestive enzymes). Lastly, she had zero good bacteria (lactobacillus and bifidobacteria), high levels of possible pathological bacteria, and yeast overgrowth.

This lab reports what is wrong and how to fix it using prescriptive and natural substances. In Lee's case, the herbs uva-ursi* and garlic were recommended to kill the bacteria and yeast. In addition, I recommended a digestive enzyme to help her body break down fats, protein, and starches more effectively. In many cases as people age, their levels of digestive enzymes decline, making it more difficult to digest everyday meals. Lastly, I suggested Lee follow a yeast-free diet for one month. The major elements of a yeast-free diet are to cut out the foods that make yeast grow like sugar, alcohol, fermented foods, and refined carbohydrates that quickly turn to sugar. Instead the foods to eat are high in protein, essential fats and fiber. A natural by-product of this diet is to lose weight, which Lee did.

Yeast Free Diet

Foods Recommended:

Meat, Fish, Chicken, Eggs

Fresh Nuts (not peanuts or pistachios which are moldy)

Fresh Fruit—two per day because of high sugar content (peeled, no moldy fruit like melon, grapes or berries).

Grains: brown rice, buckwheat, corn, wheat, millet, quinoa, spelt, oats, rye

Lots of water, green, white and red teas

Oils: flax, olive, canola or walnut

Foods to Avoid:

Sugar and all things that mean sugar i.e. honey, corn & maple syrup

Fermented foods and foods with vinegar such as condiments (ketchup, mayo, soy sauce, mustard, salad dressings)

Yeasty foods (alcohol, bread, bagels)

Commercial juices

Results

After I had worked with Lee on and off for a period of four years she had total improvement of her symptoms. She also lost weight, was able to travel to Europe, play tennis, and eat an occasional food off of her diet without any trouble. When she went back to her old eating habits, the symptoms would flare up again. This is a common problem that I see with many of my patients and have also experienced myself.

Sometimes a patient will say, "Why do I have to be on such a restrictive diet and take my supplements when my husband can eat whatever he wants?" The answer is that we all have different constitutions. Some of us have such sensitive guts and digestion that we must eat a certain way for our whole life if we want to stay healthy, be energetic, and feel good on a daily basis. That may mean giving up sugar, alcohol, and caffeine for good. I know from first-hand experience that this isn't easy, but when I or my patients feel sick after going back to a poor diet, most of us agree that it is worth it. Of course some of my patients tell me in the beginning that they will never give up sugar, caffeine, alcohol or chocolate, so we work around this and have them change what they are willing to change. Although they might not have as dramatic results as those who follow all of my recommendations, they will still be moving in the right direction. What fun is life anyway without a few small vices? As my colleague J.J. Virgin tells her patients, use the three-bite rule on foods that you can't give up. Have three bites and then throw them away. That way you will never feel deprived.

Lee's Makeover: Before

Problem: Irritable bowel, candida, poor diet	Lee had irritable bowel that was ruining her life. She had severe bowel urgency that made it difficult for her to leave the house and do the things she enjoyed.
Diet:	Lee's diet was a common Southern diet high in fat and fried foods. She also ate prepared and convenience foods and had a fair amount of sugar and alcohol. She ate little quality protein and few vegetables.
Supplements:	Lee was not taking any supplements when she first came to see me.
Exercise:	Lee loved to play tennis and tried to play 3 times a week when she was feeling well.
Stress Mgt. & Self-Care:	Lee had no formal program to relieve stress, which is usually high in patients with irritable bowel.

Lee's Makeover: After Total Wellness Program

Problem: Irritable bowel, candida, poor diet	After several tests we found Lee to have candida and other bowel abnormalities. After changing her diet and helping with these problems, she regained normal bowel function and was able to travel and play tennis again.

Diet:	I recommended that Lee reduce her meat, dairy, sugar, and alcohol consumption that was contributing to her gut inflammation and arthritis. The meal plan that I recommended was high in fiber, quality protein, and lots of water. Wheat was originally withdrawn from her diet but was able to be added back in small quantities once her digestive tract was healed.
Supplements:	Lee followed the 4 R program with many nutrients rotated in and out until her symptoms resolved. She was then on a maintenance program that included probiotics, a multi, fish oil, glucosamine, and vitamin E.
Exercise:	Once Lee felt better, she was able to go back to her regular tennis program, which improved her energy and stress level.
Stress Mgt. & Self-Care:	Lee learned relaxation exercises and how to calm herself down if she suspected a flare-up of her symptoms. Deep breathing and going back to her original food plan always seemed to work.

Cheryl's Health Makeover—Gastric Reflux, Weight-loss, Constipation, Psoriasis, Asthma

Background

When Cheryl came to see me she was highly stressed with poor health and weight-gain that had escalated over the last five years since menopause. Her doctor recommended that she see a nutritionist for weight loss and management of her gastric reflux problem. Reflux usually occurs when hydrochloric acid, which is used by the stomach for digestion, backs up into the esophagus. It can be caused by eating too many spicy or fatty foods, and consuming a diet high in alcohol, coffee, citrus fruits, chocolate, milk, and tomato based foods.

The major symptoms of gastric reflux are burning and rawness in the digestive tract, coughing and mucus in the throat. Some people get severe pains in their chest that makes them feel as though they are having a heart attack.

Cheryl was on medication for high blood pressure, asthma, and reflux. She had low energy and poor sleep quality. At 55, she was 5'6" and her weight was 185. She walked daily when the weather was good and took a multi-vitamin, vitamins C & E, calcium, and glucosomine.

For breakfast Cheryl typically ate an English muffin, toast, or cereal. Lunch consisted of a sandwich or yogurt. For dinner it was usually meat and potatoes, or a healthy choice meal. After dinner Cheryl usually got sweet cravings and chose ice cream or a frozen fruit pop. Throughout the day she drank coffee, tea, water, milk, Gatorade, and cranberry juice. In terms of stress, Cheryl had a good marriage but recently lost both of her parents. She was also worried about two of her children who had health issues.

Treatment

Diet

I recommended that Cheryl eliminate the foods mentioned above that aggravate reflux and eat small balanced meals and two snacks all with protein to keep her blood sugar stabilized and energy up. Eating small balanced meals and not eating past seven PM is very important to prevent heartburn and reflux. I asked Cheryl to increase her fiber level to 25-35 grams per day by choosing high fiber breads and cereals, and eating plenty of fruits, vegetables and legumes. I also suggested she add ground flax seeds to her cereal, salads, and yogurt since they are high in fiber and help with inflammation. This would help with both constipation and reflux and fill her up to promote healthy weight-loss.

Exercise & Stress Management

For exercise I recommended that Cheryl walk three-five times per week for at least 30 minutes and start adding strength and conditioning exercises. Since she couldn't rely on the weather always being good, Cheryl picked out a video tape that had a combination of aerobic and strength and conditioning exercises for women over 50. This would help not only with weight loss and osteoporosis prevention, but also with managing stress better. In addition, I showed Cheryl some deep breathing exercises to help her calm down when she was feeling very stressed or anxious.

Supplements

The nutritional supplements Cheryl needed were: acidophilus, aloe, a gastric repair product to help with her digestive symptoms, and a fish oil supplement to help with inflammation and psoriasis.

Results

On her follow-up visit, Cheryl reported more energy in general, improved psoriasis and no more heartburn. The constipation was also resolved and she was now drinking at least 64 ounces of water a day. Her walking had increased to four times a week and she was doing strength and conditioning exercises three times a week. In addition, the asthma improved and Cheryl no longer was coughing although she was still on maintenance doses of her medication. In about five months Cheryl reduced her weight to 165 lbs. with her goal of 150 lbs. now achievable.

Summary

I think Cheryl had underlying food sensitivities to milk and milk products that were not only aggravating her reflux but her psoriasis and asthma as well When she switched to soy milk and stopped consuming ice cream and yogurt a lot of her problems resolved. In addition, drinking more water, increasing her exercise, and adding enough fiber to alleviate constipation helped detoxify Cheryl's system. This also probably contributed to better skin quality, improved energy, and Cheryl's ability to handle stress more effectively.

Cheryl's Makeover: Before

Problem: Gastric reflux, overweight, constipation, psoriasis, asthma	Cheryl came to see me because she had so many connected problems and none of the medical treatments that she was on were helping her get better.
Diet:	Cheryl's diet had a good deal of junk food and dairy products which were making her reflux and asthma worse.
Supplements:	Cheryl was taking a multiple vitamin, vitamins C & E, calcium, and glucosomine.
Exercise:	Although Cheryl walked when she could, she wasn't on a regular schedule and only fit it in when she had extra time.
Stress Mgt. & Self-Care:	Cheryl was religious and regularly attended church and prayed. She also wrote in her journal daily and read to relax herself.

Cheryl's Makeover: After Total Wellness Program

Problem: Gastric reflux, overweight, constipation, psoriasis, asthma	After Cheryl completely changed her diet most of her symptoms went away and she lost 20 lbs. The weight loss and resolved constipation were also significant for alleviating the gastric reflux symptoms. Removing dairy products from her diet helped with the psoriasis and asthma as well.
Diet:	I recommended that Cheryl reduce her dairy, fatty, and acidic foods, as well as the sugar and tea consumption that was contributing to her gastric reflux symptoms. The meal plan that was suggested was small frequent meals that were high in fiber, with lots of vegetables, quality protein, and water.
Supplements:	Cheryl added probiotics, fish oil, and several nutrients to help heal her gut lining.

Exercise:	After starting the diet and feeling better, Cheryl began to walk regularly and also do strength and conditioning exercises with light weights. This helped with her weight loss.
Stress Mgt. & Self-Care:	Cheryl had a child with type I diabetes and was very stressed out about her condition. I taught Cheryl to breathe when she found herself thinking of the worst case scenarios. It wouldn't help her child to be anxious and would be more productive to be calm if special care was needed.

Anne's Health Makeover—Gas, Bloating, Weight-loss

Background

Anne was 45 when I first met her, and complained of gas/pressure problems nightly after dinner, post nasal drip, as well as some joint stiffness. She suspected food sensitivities and wanted to be tested. In addition, she complained of an over-active bladder, skin problems, thyroid issues which had her on Synthroid (brand name for a popular thyroid medication) for many years, and a sweet tooth, especially craving chocolate. Anne had previously attended one of my weight loss classes so her diet looked pretty good. She was already taking a multi-vitamin, calcium supplement, vitamin E, glucosamine sulfate, CoQ10, vitamin C, acidophilus, fish oil, and a cranberry supplement to help with what she considered frequent bladder infections.

Treatment

I recommended that Anne stop taking the cranberry supplement as I thought it might be contributing to a chronic cystitis (later diagnosed as interstitial cystitis which was discussed in the previous chapter). While cranberry helps with regular urinary tract infections, it increases symptoms when there is interstitial cystitis and should not be used. I also suggested Anne increase her fiber intake to 25-35 grams a day, add more water, and quality protein to snacks and meals. I urged Anne to reduce her sugar and alcohol consumption. As far as supplements go, I recommended a calcium supplement that was balanced with phosphorus, magnesium and vitamin D. These things are crucial for the absorption of the calcium and for bone health. Many times patients will use Tums or another type of calcium supplement that has just calcium, which does not do the whole job of osteoporosis prevention. I also suspected that Anne might have a magnesium deficiency. Craving chocolate could be one indication that such a deficiency exists, since chocolate is high in magnesium.

After completing a food sensitivity test we found that Anne was sensitive to 14 foods, with cow's milk, egg, almond, and brewer's yeast as the biggest offenders. I suggested that she remove all challenging foods for one month and then do a pig-out, eating high quantities of foods she was sensitive to for one day, noting any changes in symptoms. After three days of watching for symptoms, a new food could be added back and tested the same way.

Results

On our follow-up appointment Anne revealed that she had no more gas or bloating symptoms. She was able to add the foods back on a rotation basis, consuming each food no more than every third day, without any problems. Her energy was improved and she was losing weight.

Anne's Makeover: Before

Problem: Gas, weight-gain	Anne came to see me because she suspected food sensitivities. She had constant nighttime gas and bloating and couldn't identify what could be the trigger foods. She also had gained weight over the years that she couldn't lose.

Diet:	Since Anne had come to one of my classes on weight management her diet was pretty good. Her weakness was chocolate, which she craved nightly.
Supplements:	Anne was taking a multiple vitamin, vitamins C and E, fish oil, CoQ10, calcium, and glucosomine.
Exercise:	Anne tried to walk and do aerobics at the gym, but due to her hectic schedule she missed going most weeks.
Stress Mgt. & Self-Care:	Managing Anne's hectic work schedule and taking care of her children was a constant stress. Other than going out for an occasional drink with a girlfriend, Anne had no formal program to relax and take care of herself.

Anne's Makeover: After Total Wellness Program

Problem: Gas, bloating, weight-gain	Once we identified the food sensitivities and removed those foods from Anne's diet, her gas and bloating subsided. She was also able to lose weight, which she hadn't been able to do in years even though, for the most part, she was eating a healthy diet.
Diet:	Removed cow's milk, egg, almond, and brewer's yeast from Anne's diet. Otherwise she followed a basic healthy plan with plenty of vegetables, protein, fruit, and some high fiber whole grains.
Supplements:	Anne was already taking a good amount of supplements. I suggested she switch to a better multiple vitamin and calcium supplement, and stop taking the cranberry tablets.
Exercise:	Although Anne had a very busy schedule, she prioritized going to the gym three times a week for aerobics and weights and tried to do fun family activities with the kids on the week-ends.
Stress Mgt. & Self-Care:	Anne began writing in a daily journal to be in better touch with her emotions and stress triggers. This plus the exercise program helped to manage her stress better.

Like many people, Anne was suffering from food sensitivities that were resulting in gas and bloating. There are many other symptoms associated with food intolerances that most people are unaware of. The following is a partial list:

Diarrhea	Anxiety
Constipation	Bed-wetting
Gastritis	Fatigue
Malabsorption	Asthma
Weight gain	Ear infections
Acne	Interstitial cystitis
Eczema	Dark circles under the eyes
Psoriasis	Irritability
Hives	Hyperactivity
Arthritis	Headaches

If you think you or someone in your family might have some of these symptoms, consider filling out the following check list put together by Immuno Labs, one of the laboratories that does this kind of test.

If you have a lot of three's and four's in several of the areas on the chart, there is a good chance that you have food sensitivities. More information on Immuno labs and other labs that do this test can be found in the resource section.

IMMUNO HEALTH GUIDE™ INITIAL SYMPTOM CHECKLIST

Use the point scale to rate your symptoms based on how you've been feeling over the past 30 days.

0 = never or almost never have the symptom
1 = occasionally have it, effect is not severe
2 = occasionally have it, effect is severe
3 = frequently have it, effect is not severe
4 = frequently have it, effect is severe

DIGESTIVE TRACT

Nausea & vomiting
Diarrhea
Constipation
Bloated feeling
Stomach pains or cramps
Heartburn
Blood and/or mucous in stools
Total _____

EARS

Itchy ears
Ear aches, ear infections
Drainage from ear
Ringing in ears
Hearing loss
Reddening of ears
Total _____

EMOTIONS

Mood swings
Anxiety, fear, nervousness
Anger, irritability, aggressiveness
Argumentative
Frustrated, cries easily
Depression
Total_____

ENERGY & ACTIVITY

Apathy, lethargy

Attention deficit
Fatigue
Hyperactivity/restlessness
Poor physical condition
Stuttering or stammering
Slurred speech
Total_____

EYES

Watery or itchy eyes
Red, swollen, or sticky eyelids
Bags or dark circles under eyes
Blurred or tunnel vision
Total _____

HEAD

Headaches
Faintness
Dizziness
Insomnia, sleep disorder
Facial flushing
Total _____

HEART

Irregular or skipped heartbeat
Rapid or pounding heartbeat
Chest pain
Total _____

JOINTS & MUSCLES

Pains or aches in joints
Arthritis
Stiffness or limited movement
Pain or aches in muscles
Feeling of weakness or tiredness
Swollen tender joints
Growing pains in legs
Total _____

LUNGS

Chest congestion
Asthma, bronchitis
Shortness of breath
Difficulty in breathing
Persistent cough
Wheezing
Total_____

MIND

Poor memory
Difficulty completing projects
Difficulty with mathematics
Underachiever
Poor/short attention span
Confusion
Easily distracted
Difficulty making decisions
Learning disabilities
Total_____

MOUTH & THROAT

Chronic coughing
Gagging, often clearing throat
Sore throat, hoarse, loss of voice
Swollen or discolored tongue, lips
Canker sores
Itching on roof of mouth
Total_____

NOSE

Stuffy nose
Chronically red, inflamed nose
Sinus problems
Hay fever
Sneezing attacks
Excessive mucous formation
Total _____

SKIN

Acne
Itching
Hives, rash, dry skin
Hair loss
Flushing or hot flashes
Total_____

WEIGHT

Binge eating/drinking
Craving certain foods
Excessive weight

Compulsive eating
Water retention
Total _____

OTHER

Frequent illness
Frequent or urgent urination
Genital/Anal itch or discharge
Total _____

_____ **GRAND TOTAL**

5

Children's Health: Help Without Drugs for Allergies, Asthma, Ear Infections, Poor Immune & Digestive Function, ADD/ADHD, Autism

Talking about food sensitivities is a good transition into this next section of the book since so many children have problems that are tied to food allergies or sensitivities. I have seen thousands of children with everyday problems like picky eating, allergies, and asthma as well as children with complex problems like ADHD, sensory integration dysfunction, and severe autism. Most of these children have underlying digestive issues, nutrient deficiencies, allergies, or other immune system deficits.

This is a good time to explain the differences between true food allergies and food sensitivities, since many patients go to an allergist who tests them for foods and declares "no allergy." What the physician is testing in serum is the IgE immunoglobulin, the test for an immediate response allergy. An example is how my body reacts when I eat shrimp. I get the immediate responses of sneezing, itchy and watery eyes, scratchy throat, or I might break out in hives. For some people the symptoms could be as severe as a swollen tongue or a deadly anaphylactic reaction. Usually there is a genetic predisposition to the trigger foods and the reaction recurs whenever the food is eaten, no matter what the interval is between episodes. Luckily not that many people have true allergies to food; they can be outgrown, and there are usually only a few foods that would trigger this kind of response.

Food sensitivities are delayed response reactions to eating one or more foods. They can be tested by blood using IgG and other immunoglobulins that will show delayed response intolerances. The reaction can take place from two to 72 hours after eating the food(s) so it is very hard to determine which foods trigger the response. The types of symptoms are varied, as explained in the previous chapter, but in children they seem to relate particularly to behavior issues, digestion, skin, or immune problems. The most common foods that trigger a response are the foods most widely found in children's diets: milk and milk products, wheat, nuts, egg, corn, and chocolate.

The telltale signs of food allergy in children are "allergy shiners," dark circles and puffiness around the eyes. Other physical signs include chronic swollen glands, bloating, complaint of stomach ache, and frequent stuffed or runny nose. While an "allergy" is generally an immune-mediated response as a result of a protein intolerance from a given food, a "sensitivity" is usually caused by biochemical imbalance, impaired detoxification or gut functioning. Usually when these problems are addressed and the four R's that were mentioned in the previous chapter are applied, the patient is able to go back to eating the foods that they are sensitive to on a rotational basis. By rotational, I mean eating the food or associated food group every three to four days. For example, if the sensitivity is to milk products then every three or four days the patient can have cheese, milk, cream, ice cream, yogurt or butter, but never so much as to overload the system.

There are certain exceptions to this rule, particularly with children who are on the autistic spectrum. Many of them can never go back to eating products with casein, the milk protein, or gluten, the protein found in wheat, rye, barley or oats, because they are not only sensitive to it, but these proteins have peptides (protein chains) that cannot be properly broken down and cause a drug like effect in the body.

When I work with children with food sensitivities the strategy is to heal the gut and to slowly re-introduce foods over a period of three months to a year. Before the healing is complete, digestive support using enzymes and probiotics is warranted as well as anti-inflammatory nutrients and immune boosters like omega 3 & 6 oils, vitamin-C and bioflavanoids,* carotenoids,* vitamin E with selenium, and bromelain* and boswellia.*

There are many theories as to why there are so many sick children today, particularly so many diagnosed with ADHD and autism. Some people think there are environmental factors, or problems with our foods system, particularly early weaning and all of the artificial dyes, additives and chemicals in our food supply. Others feel that there are problems tied to early vaccinations with multiple vaccines such as the Measles-Mumps-Rubella(MMR) or vaccinations with preservatives like thimerosal* which may contain mercury or aluminum and be too much for an infant's developing immune system.

This is particularly a problem when the American newborn gets the first vaccination in the hospital before it develops protective micro flora of its own. The first flora that the newborn is exposed is acquired from the mother. If it is a normal vaginal birth then it will acquire acidophilus, the healthy micro flora, provided the mother has an adequate amount. If there is a c-section, which is becoming more common in the U.S., the baby will not be anointed with mom's healthy micro flora and will instead be exposed to enterobacteria such as e coli which will increase the child's chances of developing allergies or colitis later on. If mom breast-feeds in the first six months, there is a much better chance of providing her baby with healthy bacteria and a strong immune system.

Dr. Nigel Plummer, who was mentioned in the previous chapter, is leading a big clinical trial in the U.K. with approximately 3000 subjects to prove the effectiveness of probiotic organisms in the prevention of child onset sensitivities such as eczema, asthma and rhinitis.

I feel compelled to work with children and get them on the right path early. That way they don't get over medicated, potentially leading to immune system problems or worse later on. It is important to work with a pediatrician who doesn't over prescribe antibiotics for every earache or bad cold. Of course there are situations when antibiotics or other drugs are warranted and should be used.

What I am most worried about and see quite frequently in my young patients is chronic infections causing an overuse of antibiotics which not only kills the infection but also wipes out friendly protective bacteria. This can start a vicious cycle of infection. A child starts out with a small ear infection and the doctor prescribes ten days of antibiotics, which reports indicate are often not necessary, instead of trying natural treatments or taking a wait and see attitude. The drug kills the bacteria that caused the infection, and also the good germs which protect the gut and immune systems. For a viral illness—most often the case—the antibiotic has no effect on the causative organism.

According to Dr. Plummer, depending on the antibiotic used, as much as 95% of the micro flora can be eliminated with each round of antibiotics. It usually takes two-three weeks for a new colony to develop, and this new group of micro flora has a much greater amount of yeast and other antibiotic resistant organisms.

The lack of good bacteria available to crowd out the bad can now lead to a yeast overgrowth problem which compromises the integrity of the gut mucosal lining. A "leaky gut" in the intestines can develop as undigested proteins from food are absorbed in the blood stream instead of being properly digested. This can cause food sensitivities, hyperactivity or problems with attention and focus. In addition, the yeast overgrowth could cause an overall toxic state by its own penetration of toxic molecules which will weaken the immune system further, thus creating more ear infections and another vicious cycle.

There is now evidence of a connection between gut problems, neurological functioning and the immune system. Psychoneuroimmunology refers to interactions between the emotional state, nervous system, and the immune system. There is a growing body of knowledge documenting the mind's profound influence on health and disease. We know that mood affects the way we feel on a daily basis and that positive imagery can potentially reverse disease.

When I work with children I often see these connections. A child will come in with diarrhea, hyperactivity, mood swings, and a poorly functioning immune system that is manifested by frequent infections requiring treatment with antibiotics. Once we implement the 4-R recovery program described in the previous chapter to heal the gut, the immune system improves, the child is not frequently getting sick any more, and the moody and hyperactive behavior lessens. If the child is able to stay off the antibiotics than the good results will last a long time. Sometimes, however, the need for antibiotics arises (as in the case of lyme disease, which is seen frequently in the Northeast, or strep throat) and the cycle begins again.

We also know that stress has a big role in the cause of diseases. Stress in children can be a problem and should not be overlooked. Divorce is on the rise, and many households have both parents working. There are also displays of violence on the nightly news, and in movies, television and video games. School is more challenging and children are bombarded with a myriad of after-school programs to choose from. Where is the down time, and how do children de-stress?

Stress impacts the immune system negatively. It increases adrenal gland hormones. This in turn inhibits white blood cell formation and causes the thymus gland to shrink (a key gland for fighting off viral infections).

Another tie-in is possible nutritional deficiencies that can affect the emotional state and immunity. Many kids with learning problems and associated self-esteem issues are now being labeled with depression. Some studies now show depression to be associated with functional immune decrements and immune over-activation.

There is also a strong connection between children with poor immune and digestive functions. I discussed earlier the problem of chronic yeast overgrowth problems from antibiotic over-use causing leaky gut syndrome and subsequent nutrient malabsorption. Inadequate nutrient intake or absorption could be one causative factor for irritable bowel, colitis or crohn's disease. Another possible factor is constipation problems leading to toxic waste being stored in the body which may decrease immune function.

Bearing this in mind, and understanding that there are also environmental factors like outdoor/indoor pollutants, pesticides, food and water chemicals that can wreak havoc on the immune system, what are concerned parents to do? The key is to try to prevent problems in the first place. Would a child without underlying immune problems develop allergies, asthma or learning disabilities if he or she was not genetically predisposed? I would suspect the answer to be no. Even if your child is not prone to getting infections, following these basic guidelines will help make the immune system stronger.

Guidelines for All Children

1. Decrease or remove sugary and processed foods like candy, soda, refined grain products, and foods with dyes, colors or preservatives. Eliminate all trans fats from the diet. These altered fats are dangerous and may create an essential fatty acid balance, leading to learning disabilities, allergies and asthma.

2. Ensure your child is getting enough whole, organic foods such as fresh fruits and vegetables, unprocessed complex carbohydrates (like high fiber cereal, sprouted wheat bread, and beans), quality protein, and nuts and seeds.

3. Make sure your child consumes enough pure water. I recommend 24 to 48 oz., depending on the weight of the child. This helps prevent dehydration and is particularly important for children who tend to be constipated. If your child is consuming mostly juice, it should be watered down to no more than a third of

a glass of juice to two thirds water. This will get them used to the taste.

4. After decreasing your child's intake of processed foods, give him/her an all natural multi-vitamin and mineral supplement. It works best to give these vitamins with meals in divided doses to keep the nutrients in the blood stream throughout the day. Most children do not get enough minerals on a daily basis from the food they eat so the multi gives insurance that your child will get what is lacking in the diet.

5. If your child is getting sick give him/her the herbs echinacea,* garlic, and astragalus,* as well as vitamin C, and carrot juice. From my experience I have found these to boost the immune system and help prevent or shorten the duration of colds and other viral infections.

6. If the child has an ear infection, warm garlic and mullein oil in the ear canal for a week can help. The garlic kills the infection and fights pain, and the mullein oil* helps drain the fluid. If you catch the infection late and your child needs antibiotics, make sure to use a probiotics supplement during the treatment and for at least a week afterwards. This will replenish the good flora in the intestines and reduce the chance of a yeast overgrowth. Note that the probiotic supplement should be taken several hours away from the antibiotic and with food so that the stomach acid will be used to digest the meal and will not inhibit the probiotic supplement from getting into the intestines.

Additional Steps for Parents with Kids With Allergies, Asthma, ADHD, Autistic Spectrum

7. If you suspect that your child has food sensitivities, find a professional to work with who can help identify these intolerances. Many kids with learning problems and chronic ear infections have

milk or wheat sensitivities. Other common culprits are peanuts, corn, eggs, yeast or soy, and foods with artificial colors or preservatives. Sensitivities worsen over time when children often eat the same foods daily.

8. Investigate the possibility of yeast overgrowth. Yeast problems can have an impact on behavior and can weaken the immune system. A stool or urine test by the right lab can determine if this is a problem.

9. Another test that can be a good diagnostic tool is hair mineral/ toxic metal screening. I often see children with depressed levels of chromium, iron, magnesium, and zinc, and elevated levels of aluminum, copper, mercury, and lead who are prone to ADHD and other illnesses. When the child is exposed to lead, it will show up in the blood for around 30 days and then migrate to cells and tissues where a blood test will no longer pick it up. The hair analysis will reflect the biochemistry of the patient over time, including the mineral and metal levels. It should be mentioned that the most highly mercury toxic individuals often have mercury lodged in their organs and it will not show up in the hair. The best way to test for mercury toxicity, according to expert Dr. Dietrich Kinghart, is to get a baseline hair test. If the test shows no elevated mercury but there is a suspicion that there is a problem, as with many autistic children, Klinghart recommends treating the child with natural mercury binders like cilantro and chlorella. After 6 weeks of treatment another hair test should be done. If it shows no mercury at this point there is probably none to worry about. If it shows elevated mercury then it means it is being pulled out and eliminated. The process should continue and follow a bell curve with mercury at a baseline of zero or at a low level, then going up, peaking and finally going down and to zero. This type of testing is validated by the clinical research of Dr. Amy Holmes who published a piece in Toxicology, 2003 which associated the amount of mercury in birth hair with the severity of autism. According to her

research the children with the least amount of mercury in their hair were the most autistic. However they carry a higher mercury body burden than control children because they are unable to effectively detoxify this neurotoxin and also have a genetic predisposition causing retention toxicity. It is also worthy to note in the same work by Dr. Holmes that the children who showed the highest amount of mercury in their hair at birth were children whose mothers had a large number of amalgam fillings.

10. For kids that are prone to infections and allergies, I recommend a daily vitamin C supplement to boost the immune system. Vitamin C builds white blood cells to prevent viruses and ear infections, and acts as a natural antihistamine. It should be given in divided doses throughout the day since the body uses what it needs and gets rid of the rest. If too much is given then the only real side effect is loose stools.

11. Many children can benefit from taking essential fatty acids such as EPA, DHA, and GLA. These essential fatty acids can help with brain development, neurological functioning as well as skin problems like eczema. Some companies that make baby formula are now adding DHA as an ingredient since there is evidence that it can help the developing brain.

12. If your child has frequent ear infections, allergies or asthma symptoms, try doing a three week elimination of all milk products. Dairy products are mucus forming and inflammatory which makes these conditions worse. There is a lot of controversy over the merits of giving children cow's milk since we are the only species that drinks another species' milk. If you give your child milk-based products, make sure they are organic and do not have antibiotics or growth hormones. There are many alternative food sources for calcium which are mentioned in chapter 9, or you can give your child a calcium/magnesium supplement to ensure there are enough of these important minerals for growth and bone health. Calcium

and magnesium also have a calming effect on children and help them to sleep better.

Let's review a few makeover examples to tie together how these problems manifest in children and what can be done about them.

Allison's Health Makeover—ADHD, Poor Digestion, Sensory Integration, and Food Sensitivities

Background

Alison was two ½ years old when she first came to see me. She was normal at birth, but after having her first round of immunizations at two months of age, she developed chronic diarrhea with blood and mucus in the stool. When I first met Alison, she was hyperactive with poor attention span, and was suspected of being somewhere on the autistic spectrum although she had good eye contact and no problems speaking. Her parents wanted help with the diet and digestive issues foremost. Recently Alison had been to a pediatric gastroenterologist who did several tests and found no problems. She also went to an allergy specialist at Columbia Presbyterian Medical Center in New York City who stated in his letter to the referring doctor, "allergy does not contribute to Alison's problems," after doing the radioallergosorbent test (RAST) using serum IgE for egg, milk, tuna, tomato, apple, cheddar cheese, mold, wheat, casein, peanut, walnut, and dust mites.

During my first visit with Alison and her parents, it was clear that she (and they) were in distress. She couldn't sit still, had large allergy shiners under her eyes, and her color was poor, a symptom which usually reflects a malfunctioning immune system. Her parents confirmed this by telling me Alison had chronic congestion, sore throats, cough, and a drippy nose.

Treatment

My approach was first to work on Alison's diet. We removed the sweets and preservatives and added protein with each meal and snack to help stabilize blood sugar, thereby reducing her hyperactivity and irritability. The next step was to heal the digestive tract by using the 4R principle—first, remove foods she was sensitive to as well as any germs, bad bacteria or toxic metals using anti-fungal herbs and natural heavy metal chelators. Next re-introduce the digestive system with good bacteria and digestive enzymes. Then replace the diet with healthy non-processed foods, vitamins, minerals, and essential fatty acids. Lastly, repair the gut lining with glutamine,* DGL,* aloe leaf,* MSM,* slippery elm,* and marshmallow root.*

The next steps were improving Alison's immune system, helping with her sensory issues, and facilitating her liver detoxification. Normally I like to handle digestive problems first before moving on. In this case the immune system was functioning so poorly, I needed to make some recommendations to keep her from getting sick and on antibiotics in the future.

The family decided to test the following: stool using the specialized laboratory mentioned earlier, IgG food sensitivities, hair mineral/toxic metals, and urine organic acids to find inborn errors in metabolism and assess her detoxification pathways.

Alison's IgG food sensitivity test revealed that she was "very" sensitive to nine foods. The most significant were eggs, milk products, and sugar. Her stool test revealed undigested food and mucus, no beneficial bacteria and possibly bad bacteria. The hair test showed low calcium and magnesium levels (the relaxing or quieting minerals), high sodium and potassium (which may indicate high adrenal and cortisol levels—the stress indicators), low zinc and elevated aluminum, which both have to do with attention, focus, and memory problems. Last, the urine test revealed yeast metabolites and other nutritional deficiencies.

You may be wondering why there was a discrepancy with the tests that were done by Alison's doctors. This is best answered by looking at the differences between traditional and alternative medicine. Using an IgE antibody to test for immediate response food allergies is the standard test done by doctors and allergists. Many naturopaths and nutritionists will also check for food sensitivities, a delayed response, through other antibodies as well, as explained before. The hair test, although widely used by the police force for drug and forensic testing, is not generally accepted in the traditional medical community. Many in natural medicine feel it is one of the best overall markers of nutritional status because unlike blood, which reveals just a day at a time, the hair reflects the last six months of your life. Some of the stool and urine tests may be more acceptable by conventional doctors, but there may be differences in the labs used and the extensiveness of the test which may yield different results.

Results

Over the next year and a half I worked closely with Alison's parents focusing on her diet, removing the foods she was sensitive to, adding protein and essential fats, and rotating various nutrients in and out to help heal her gut, build her immune system, and improve the underlying toxicity problems. The result is a child with normal bowel function, improved immune system, better concentration and focus, and somewhat improved hyperactivity. We are continuing to work on this and her remaining sensory issues, and I am optimistic about Alison's chances of enrolling in a mainstream kindergarten program when the time comes.

Alison's Makeover: Before

Problem: ADHD, loose stools, sensory issues, food sensitivities	Alison had chronic diarrhea since two months of age. She was hyperactive with a short attention span. She had large allergy shiners under her eyes and looked like a "typical allergy kid." She also had poor color and was constantly sick.

Diet:	Alison's diet had too much sugar and refined carbohydrates as well as artificial colors and preservatives. She did not have protein for breakfast or for lunch and consumed too much dairy.
Supplements:	The prescribed children's multi with fluoride was being used.
Exercise:	Alison was very active and was getting occupational therapy.
Stress Mgt. & Self-Care:	The parents were doing behavior management therapy with Alison, but it didn't seem to be helping.

Alison's Makeover: After Total Wellness Program

Problem: ADHD, loose stools, sensory issues, food sensitivities	Once we identified the food sensitivities and removed those foods from Alison's diet her diarrhea subsided. We built up her immune system by cutting out sugar and refined foods and used a variety of supplements to give her the nutrienst that she was deficient in.
Diet:	Removed cow's milk, egg, and sugar from Alison's diet. We gave her small frequent meals with some protein in each to help keep her blood sugar and moods stable.
Supplements:	We used a variety of nutrients to help with Alison's digestive function. Most of these were rotated and used on a short term basis. To help with Alison's focus and attention problems I recommended a product that was designed to help with cognitive and neurotransmitter function.
Exercise:	Alison continued to participate in a lot of activities in pre-school and in her occupational therapy sessions. Her parents also did other sensory exercises with her throughout the day.
Stress Mgt. & Self-Care:	We used the Bach flower rescue remedy when Alison was having a tantrum and could not stop herself or when she could not wind down enough to go to sleep. I also recommended Epsom salt baths at night and a calcium magnesium supplement to help her fall asleep easier.

Bobby's Health Makeover—Poorly Functioning Immune System, and Chronic Strep Throat

Background

Bobby was seven years old when he came to see me. He had chronic strep throat; 12 times in the last two years, with one incident taking three courses of antibiotics to clear up. In addition, he had moderate irritability, tantrums, low muscle tone, fatigue, and some food allergies. His parents wanted a healthier child with a vitamin regimen to keep him off of antibiotics in the future.

Although I don't see chronic strep throat that often, the treatment is similar to chronic ear infections, colds, and runny noses. In all of these cases the problem is clearly a poorly functioning immune system. The key is to find any nutritional deficiencies, detoxification or digestive issues that are contributing to the problem, fix those, and at the same time build up a strong defense to prevent further infections.

When I looked at Bobby's diet it was like most children's—low protein and high carbohydrate, especially not enough protein for breakfast. He was consuming Eggo chocolate chip waffles every morning for breakfast with a mid-morning snack of either pretzels or a cereal bar. Although Bobby was getting some protein with lunch and dinner, which is better than most kids I see, his vegetable intake consisted of romaine lettuce and baby corn.

Treatment

I asked Bobby's parents to change his breakfast and snacks to include more protein to help with blood sugar balance, muscle tone, energy and immune system health. Since he was allergic to nuts we couldn't use nuts or nut butters which make good snacks for kids. I asked his mother to give Bobby eggs, a protein drink, or switch to whole grain soy flax waffles which have protein, healthy fat, and fiber to balance out the carbohydrates for breakfast. For snacks we switched to soy chips, fruit and cheese, or turkey slices rolled up with mustard. At the end of this chapter I include lunch and snack examples for children to give you some idea of how to get away from the junky snacks sold at school which are full of sugar and hydrogenated oils.

Bobby started on supplements to boost his immune system: a children's multi-vitamin and mineral complex, garlic, mixed carotenoids, EPA/DHA, and vitamin C. We also did a hair mineral/toxic metal screening and an IgG food sensitivity test. I suspected that since Bobby already had some known food allergies, he might have some sensitivities as well that could be degrading his immune system. The parents opted to start with just the toxic metal/mineral screening.

The test revealed high copper/low zinc, low sodium and potassium, and elevated aluminum. We then added zinc to Bobby's supplement list to bring his levels up. Zinc is an important mineral for immune health but should not be given in high doses for an extended period of time. Picky eating is often a sign of zinc deficiency. There is documented evidence that some forms of anorexia nervosa can actually be caused by zinc deficiencies. I recommend giving children zinc in a liquid form. When you give a deficient child the liquid zinc it should taste just like water initially. As it begins to build back up in the body, there is a metallic taste. If the liquid drops are taken in water a zinc deficient child usually will not taste them in the beginning. When the child later refuses to drink the water with zinc because of bad taste, you know the levels are back to normal and the drops are no longer needed. I also gave Bobby's parents a list of foods high in potassium, and recommended a weekly Epsom salt bath, which aids in detoxification and improves sodium levels.

Results

Bobby has not had strep throat since our first visit over seven months ago. He did get one cold. His mother added echinacea, astragalus, and carrot juice to the vitamin C and garlic that he was already taking and the cold passed quickly. Bobby is now eating a more varied diet including a variety of vegetables sautéed with garlic and olive oil. He also has more stamina and energy.

Bobby's Makeover: Before

Problem: Poorly functioning immune system, chronic strep throat	Bobby had strep throat 12 times in a two-year period and he was becoming resistant to the standard antibiotic treatments. His mother was looking for an alternative to build his immune system and make him stronger.
Diet:	Bobby's diet was low protein and high carbohydrate. He consumed a fair amount of sugar and artificial dyes and colors. He ate few vegetables and an occasional fruit.
Supplements:	Bobby was taking a high sugar children's chewable multi vitamin.
Exercise:	Energy was an issue for Bobby so he didn't run around as much as other children his age.
Stress Mgt. & Self-Care:	Stress did not seem to be a major factor but there was the recent death of a grandparent that might have been the trigger for Bobby's initial strep throat episode.

Bobby's Makeover: After Total Wellness Program

Problem: Poorly functioning immune system, chronic strep throat	Bobby had no more strep throat episodes. He felt much better and had more energy for sports. He had one cold in the year that I followed him and his family.
Diet:	Bobby's diet was much improved. He began eating vegetables with garlic and olive oil regularly. He started the morning with either a protein drink or eggs and had protein throughout the day. He reduced his sugar intake from junky foods and began eating fruit every day.

Supplements:	Initially Bobby was on a lot of vitamins to build his immune system back up and make him stronger. He now is on a good all natural multivitamin and vitamin C, and takes garlic, astragalus, and zinc as needed to boost his immune system.
Exercise:	Energy is no longer an issue for Bobby who is involved in several organized sport activities.
Stress Mgt. & Self-Care:	Bobby's parents discussed the loss of his grandparent with him and relieved his fears, assuring him that they were going to be around for a long while.

Peter's Health Makeover—Allergies, Asthma, Behavior Problems, Sensory Issues, and Chronic Stomach Ache

Background

Peter was four when he first came to see me. His mother's primary concern was his high level of activity and inability to sit and attend. He also showed signs of sensory issues, no sense of personal space, and poor balance.

His diet was mostly carbohydrate and dairy with some fruit and protein sprinkled in. Peter frequently complained of stomach aches, and his bowel movements were usually mushy. He was on allergy medicine for a chronic cough and congestion and had been on antibiotics only once.

Treatment

My recommendations started with Peter's diet. When a child has chronic allergies and asthma the amount of dairy consumed should be evaluated since it is mucus forming and increases inflammation. This child was consuming around 6 servings a day. I requested that Peter cut back on dairy products and check to see if he had food sensitivities that could be adding to his problems. I recommended more protein with each meal, less sugar, and some fruits and vegetables to balance out his diet. In terms of vitamins, I suggested a natural complete multi-vitamin and mineral supplement, a chewable vitamin C, and alfalfa. Vitamin C and alfalfa are natural antihistamines that help with coughing and congestion.

When we got back Peter's tests, he was found to be low in minerals across the board and sensitive to 31 foods including milk, eggs, wheat, banana and cheese. His digestive test revealed bad bacteria and not enough good flora in his intestines. When a child is sensitive to so many foods there is most likely a "leaky gut" situation. His mother removed all of the high reactive foods except wheat to start (she thought it would be too much to do at once) and added some acido-philus and Saccharomyces Boulardi* to help with the digestive issues.

Saccharomyces Boulardi provides healthy bacteria to get rid of a lot of the unfriendly germs in the digestive system and helps restore normal gut flora. It is particularly useful when there are loose stools or a leaky gut. I recommended a digestive enzyme in the short-term, to help Peter digest wheat. I also added zinc, calcium/magnesium, flax oil and a product called Bio-Focus which is described in the resource section to help with attention and focus.

Results

After following the above program for about a month, Peter's allergy/asthma symptoms were much better and his stools were normal. Peter was doing well in school with better attention and behavior. On our next appointment we planned to start Peter on a gluten-free diet to see if he could achieve further improvements. Gluten grains consist of wheat, barley, rye, and oats.

Peter's Makeover: Before

Problem: Allergies, asthma, behavior problems, sensory issues, chronic stomach ache	Peter had trouble sitting still and other behavior problems. He always had a runny nose and often complained of stomach aches. He had mushy daily bowel movements. He was getting occupational therapy for some sensory issues.
Diet:	Peter's diet was mostly carbohydrates and dairy with some fruit and protein sprinkled in. He ate no vegetables.
Supplements:	He took no supplements but took daily allergy medication.
Exercise:	Peter was a high energy kid but didn't participate in enough organized sports activities.
Stress Mgt. & Self-Care:	It is hard to evaluate the level of stress that a child undergoes. Peter had trouble sleeping which could be an indication that there was something bothering him. It can also be a result of food allergies or nutritional deficiencies which we discovered Peter had.

Peter's Makeover: After Total Wellness Program

Problem: Allergies, asthma, behavior problems, sensory issues, chronic stomach ache	After changing Peter's diet and giving him some supplements to help with his attention and behavior issues he was more focused and doing better in school and at home. Once we identified his food sensitivities and removed those foods from the diet, most of Peter's allergy and asthma symptoms subsided. He still needs to use his inhaler occasionally. Peter now has normal bowel movements and has shown a lot of improvement in his sensory issues.
Diet:	Peter's diet was changed to remove dairy for a trial and his mother continued because his allergies and asthma symptoms were so much better. He also consumed more protein, less sugar, and more fruits and vegetables.
Supplements:	I recommended a chewable multi and vitamin C. Peter also used alfalfa as a natural decongestant and nutrients to help with his attention and behavior.

Exercise:	More formalized exercise was added to Peter's schedule through team sports. This helped him to build self-esteem and to improve his socialization skills.
Stress Mgt. & Self-Care:	Peter's sleep improved after he changed his diet and began taking supplements. His behavior improved and he seemed to have less internal stress.

Summary

If there is a problem with allergies, low immune function, ADHD, or Autistic Spectrum Disorder the diet, digestive, and neurological functioning all play key roles.

Children with Allergies and Asthma

It is very important to avoid milk products, dyes, sulfites and any foods that the child is sensitive to. The supplements that seem to be most helpful are vitamin C with bioflavanoids, vitamin E, garlic, and mixed carotenoids (the antioxidants normally found in yellow, orange, red, and green vegetables). According to a study recently published in the *American Journal of Epidemiology,* dietary deficiencies of the antioxidant vitamins A, C, E, and the carotenoids, have been linked to the presence and severity of asthma. This study was conducted in the United States between 1988 and 1994 and includes over four thousand children between the ages of six-17 years old.

Children with ADHD, Sensory Integration Dysfunction and Autistic Spectrum Disorders

It is important to do mineral/toxic metal analysis through hair or urine. Food sensitivity tests, and stool tests for digestive abnormalities are also important, especially if the child has a history of frequent antibiotic usage. It is common for many of these children to be low in the minerals zinc, chromium, magnesium and selenium. In fact, cities that have the lowest amounts of selenium detected in the soil seem to have the highest clusters of autism diagnosed. This could just be a coincidence, but as more is learned it is best to ensure a proper diet is followed and nutritional supplements used when needed.

Many of these children are sensitive to gluten (the protein found in wheat, barley, rye and oats) and casein (the milk protein) and do much better when they eliminate these foods and others that they are sensitive to.

They do especially well on high protein lower carbohydrate diets with plenty of essential fatty acids from flax or fish oils, either in their diets or through supplements. Digestive enzymes, acidophilus, and bifidobacteria for proper gut functioning, and natural or prescriptive antifungals to eliminate yeast overgrowths may also be needed. The following nutrients seem to be most important: B vitamins, especially B6 and B12 which help with neurological functioning; zinc which helps with immune system function, picky eating and concentration; calcium and magnesium, which have a calming effect; lecithin and ginkgo biloba* for memory; and L-tyrosine*, and other amino acids for mood stabilization, and to overcome depression.

Picking the right supplements should be individualized based on the symptoms and needs of the child. There are several companies that make complete nutritional product formulas that are palatable for small children who cannot swallow pills. You can find out more about them in the resource section.

Exercise & Stress Management

Aerobic exercise and stress management techniques are essential components in any wellness program for children. In fact, lack of exercise may be more of a factor in childhood obesity than diet. It is recommended that children should have some form of physical activity every day, but at least three times a week there should be something more organized like swimming, a running sport like soccer, or a jumping sport like gymnastics or karate.

With ADHD or autistic spectrum children this is even more important, even though many of them are already working with physical and occupational therapists where activity is an important part of their treatments. Some of these kids are very high energy and some are very low energy, but in either case the activity helps get the blood pumping to circulate nutrients to the cells and organs. It also helps in the detoxification process.

Stress management for children can be somewhat difficult since many of them cannot sit and attend for very long. Behavior therapy can work for older, more connected kids, but for younger children I like art or music therapy. I have seen many young children work well with clay.

For older kids who can focus and concentrate, meditation, yoga, and simple breathing exercises can be effective. An easy breathing technique that can be taught to any child is to breathe in for five counts and on the out breath say the words "I am calm."

As part of a program to calm or support emotional or mental energies, Bach Flower remedies can be considered. These remedies were developed in the early 1900's by Dr. Bach, a Physician and Homoeopath. They are prepared from non-poisonous wild flowers, for the purpose of achieving balance between the mind, body and spirit. Bach flower remedies work by gently correcting the emotional upsets that give rise to physical symptoms or delay recovery from an illness. They can be rubbed on the skin or taken in drop form under the tongue and are safe, non-addicting and gentle, making them excellent remedies for children.

The most popular Bach Flower is called Rescue Remedy. This remedy can be given to a child during a temper tantrum, or for sleep problems, or nervousness. I keep it in my car along with Arnica (a homeopathic remedy for bruises, sprains and muscle pains) in case of emergencies. There is usually a calming effect in a couple of minutes. There are 38 other remedies used for different emotional or mental conditions such as: mimulus or cherry plum for bedwetting due to nerves, clematis for day-dreaming, vervain for hyperactivity and restless nights, and aspen for hypersensitivity. Bach Flower remedies can be found at most health food stores.

Healthy Lunch and Snack Ideas

The final section in this chapter gives healthy lunch and snack suggestions and can be used as a guideline to help your children and family make healthier meal choices. When better alternatives are available instead of the junk food that kids are inundated with from T.V., school, etc.—children will eat them.

A perfect example of this was an effort I led several years ago at my daughter's elementary school. For one week we removed all snacks with corn syrup and hydrogenated oils and brought in daily healthy alternatives that were available for no charge in the lunch room. In addition, we sent home nightly information packets for parents on creating healthier meals and had fun class room games to show children how to read labels and pick healthy snacks. We surveyed parents, teachers, and children at the end of the week. Most of the people who took the survey were very pleased with the program. When we tried to make permanent changes in the cafeteria, however, we were told "no" by school administration because there was a contract to fulfill with a vendor and the school would lose money if they didn't sell the junk food. It was disappointing to know that the program wouldn't have a longer tenure, but satisfying to know that we had a significant impact on many children who were now more label reading savvy than their parents.

If you improve your children's diet, it is crucial to set an example for them by making better choices yourself. Some of my patients plan their children's meals well, but are so busy they hardly eat themselves, just picking during the day or finishing everybody's left overs. I explain to them that they have to take care of themselves first, or they won't be well enough to help their children.

If one member of the family has to go on a special diet, it works well to have support from the whole family. It is amazing how much better everyone feels when they reduce or eliminate refined white flour products and food that is processed with artificial colors or dyes, and high sugar content!

Healthy Meal Alternatives

Lunch Suggestions

- Leftover baked turkey or chicken on wholegrain bread with apple slices

- Applegate or similar nitrate-free ham, turkey, salami, with slice of cheese and mustard on a whole grain roll with soy chips

- Tuna sandwich or tuna burger (simply mold a mixture of tuna & low fat mayo into a patty and brown in non-stick skillet) served in a whole wheat pita with carrot sticks

- Natural peanut butter or almond butter and all-fruit spread on whole grain bread and cucumbers and celery sticks with salad dressing to dip

- Chicken or egg salad with low-fat canola oil mayo on whole wheat bread with grapes and carrot sticks

- Pizza sauce and reduced fat mozzarella cheese on a whole wheat pita & small spinach salad

- Bean burrito using vegetarian refried beans, shredded reduced fat cheese on a whole wheat tortilla. Serve with baked or non-hydrogenated corn chips and salsa

- Nitrate-free regular, turkey or soy hotdog on whole wheat bun, with fresh fruit

- Hamburger, turkey burger, or veggie burger on whole wheat bun with lettuce, tomato, cole slaw, and pickles

- Chicken, turkey, beef, or bean soup cooked with veggies and brown rice, served with a side salad and whole wheat bread

- Salad for lunch with chicken, turkey, or tuna on top with whole grain roll

- Salad with goat cheese, pear and sprinkled walnuts on top with whole grain roll

Healthy Beverages: water, skim milk, flavored seltzer water

Healthy Snacks

- Raw almonds (even low sugar chocolate or carob covered)

- Fresh fruit with low-fat cheese

- Baked or non-hydrogenated corn chips and salsa

- Raw veggies and hummus

- A hard boiled egg

- Mixture of raw nuts such as almonds, walnuts, or cashews, and dried fruit, or store bought trail mix

- Soy chips—comes in many tasty flavors, loaded with protein and low carb

- Your favorite protein bar

- Make your own Peanut Butter Chocolate Chip Bar (Good for older kids and the child in all of us)

     - use 10 tbs. protein powder (buy a low sugar variety)

     - one cup quick cooking or old-fashioned oats, uncooked

- one cup rice crispies

- one cup peanut or almond butter

- 3/4 cup honey

- 2.5 tsp. vanilla flavor extract

- 2/3 cup chocolate chips

1. Combine oats, protein, and rice crispies in large bowl and set aside

2. Bring honey to a boil on stovetop. Remove from heat and stir in peanut butter and vanilla until smooth

3. Immediately add honey mixture to dry mix until well incorporated

4. Refrigerate for 20-25 minutes

5. Stir in chocolate chips and press into 8x8 square inch pan

6. Refrigerate approximately 20 minutes or until firm

7. Cut into 12 bars and serve

8. Make extra and freeze

PART III

*An Anti-Aging Program
for Everyone to Follow*

The previous chapters and makeover examples provided information to help you and your family with specific health problems. But what if you are currently experiencing general good health and want to continue along that path with a sharp mind, healthy immune system, and good energy and vitality for the rest of your life. The following chapters are general guidelines to help you live your life to the fullest potential.

6

Detoxify Your Body

Detoxification is the process of neutralizing and eliminating toxins and waste from the body. There are many bodily processes involved in detoxification; the most notable are those performed by the liver, intestines, kidneys, and blood.

Our bodies are bombarded with chemicals, toxins and heavy metals from the air that we breathe, the food and water we take in, and many other things we are exposed to from the environment. Since World War II industrialized countries use and pass on thousands of chemicals. The by-products of these chemicals reach us in many ways. Some people use daily prescription or over-the-counter drugs, smoke, and drink alcohol, putting themselves at a higher risk for toxicity. Even those who don't often use products with chemicals on their skin, hair, and nails and eat foods sprayed with pesticides or injected with drugs. All of these chemicals are either ingested or absorbed through our skin or bronchial passages. The toxins in these products need to be neutralized and excreted. If not they will get stored in our fat cells over time and lead to premature aging and disease. The best way to ensure proper detoxification is to do the following:

- Step 1: First, reduce exposure to toxins in the first place. You could stop coloring your hair, polishing your nails, and using antiperspirants with aluminum in them. If you don't want to go that far, then you can buy organic foods and drink purified water. Using natural cleaning and laundry products reduces the chemicals that you and your family are exposed to, and helps the environment as well. If there is anyone in your house with asthma or allergies, using these natural products is particularly important. Anyone who smokes knows that quitting is an excellent place to start.

- Step 2: Eat foods that aid detoxification such as fruits, vegetables, whole grains and legumes high in fiber. According to *The Encyclopedia of Natural Medicine*, by Michael Murray, N.D. and Joseph Pizzorno, N.D., the sulfation system is important for detoxifying several drugs, food additives, and especially toxins from intestinal bacteria and the environment. Foods high in sulfur are onions, garlic, and brussell sprouts.

- Step 3: Avoid or reduce alcohol. It taxes the liver, especially if you have had hepatitis or suspect liver dysfunction.

- Step 4: Avoid fatty foods, hydrogenated or partially hydrogenated oils, caffeine, and foods with high sugar content. All of these put extra work on the adrenal glands and negatively impact the immune system.

- Step 5: Drink at least 64 ounces of water a day to help flush toxins through the bowels and kidneys. For some people a better rule of thumb is to drink water equivalent (in ounces) to half of your body weight.

- Step 6: Get plenty of exercise. As I mentioned earlier, exercise stimulates blood circulation, which helps in all bodily functions including digestion and elimination.

- Step 7: Consider seasonal fasting. Some patients benefit by doing a three day juice fast using fresh organic vegetables and fruits and plenty of water at the beginning of every season. One popular juicing combination is carrot, beet, and apple, which improves immune, liver and gallbladder functions. Fasting allows the body to rest and eliminate toxins. The energy that is normally used for digestion is utilized to heal the gut and liver instead. I usually recommend fasting for healthy individuals who want to increase their energy or jump start a weight loss program. If there is a real toxic overload problem or serious illness you should work with a qualified health care practitioner before doing any fasting, as your body may not be able to handle the side effects from rapid detoxification.

- Step 8: Consider supplementing with the following detoxifying nutrients: vitamin C, B-complex, sulfur-containing amino acids like methionine,* choline,* cysteine,* and taurine,* and herbs like milk thistle,* and dandelion root.* It is also important to support the digestive system with probiotics and bile acids to help the gallbladder and intestines remove toxins. There are many complete formulas that have a lot of these nutrients in one supplement.

- Step 9: Enjoy 10-15 minutes in a sauna or steam room, three times a week. This is a great way to open your pores and remove toxins through your sweat and skin. If you don't have access to these amenities, you could take a bath using one cup of Epsom salts, several times a week. The magnesium sulfate opens up another pathway for detoxification and is also very relaxing and good for sore muscles or period cramps. Vigorous exercise also promotes sweating and eliminating toxins.

There are some very good books that go into much greater detail on the topic of detoxification. One that I like in particular is *Detoxification and Healing* by Dr. Sidney Baker, who is a leader in integrative medicine and well-known for his pioneering work with autistic spectrum children.

7

Build a Strong Immune System

Building a healthy immune system was discussed earlier in the children's health section. Many of the same rules apply for adults with a few minor additions. There are several steps.

Step 1: Life Style Practices

Eliminate unhealthy practices such as smoking, heavy drinking or using any recreational drugs. Even over the counter drugs like aspirin, non steroidal anti-inflammatory drugs (NSAIDS), allergy medication, etc., should not be overused due to their potentially negative impact on the liver and gastrointestinal tract. One recent study on the safety of NSAIDS concluded that when consumed at a low to medium dose, there are between two and three adverse gastrointestinal events per thousand patients per year. Long term or heavier usage (even in children with juvenile arthritis) may result in serious GI bleeding, increased risk for gastric ulceration, and increased gut permeability.

If you are on prescriptive medication for blood pressure regulation or statins for cholesterol management there is a chance that you might be able to reduce or get off of these drugs with dietary modifications, exercise, stress management, and other natural supplements. Please do not reduce or go off of any medication on your own without working closely with your doctor.

Step 2: Nutrition & Body Weight

The second set of recommendations is to eat for nutrition and control of your body weight. There is a growing body of research that shows that caloric restriction boosts the immune system and leads to a longer, healthier life. It is fine to eat foods like pizza or ice cream occasionally, but they should be special treats, not staples in the diet. Awhile ago I read an article in the *Wall Street Journal* where they interviewed the CEO of PepsiCo regarding his views on the obesity epidemic in children. He said that soda and snack foods like Fritos are special occasion foods that should not be part of the daily diet. Pepsico is currently working on healthier snack food alternatives without hydrogenated oils.

The diet should consist of three balanced meals and two snacks. The bulk of the diet should come from unprocessed protein, fresh fruits and vegetables, beans, nuts and seeds, and a small amount of fibrous whole grains, and healthy oils. These foods contain plenty of essential nutrients, antioxidants, bioflavanoids, and carotenoids, all important for healthy immune function. The following chart gives you information on how much of these nutrients you can get from certain foods. The diet should be low in saturated fats, hydrogenated oils, sugar, alcohol, and processed foods. As was stated earlier, getting at least 48-64 ounces of water a day is recommended to keep you properly hydrated and the detoxification pathways working efficiently.

Antioxidants in Common Foods

Vitamin E (IU)

Wheat germ oil (Tbsp.) 20.3
Total Cereal, Gen. Mills (cup) 20
Product 19, Kellogg's (cup) 20
Sunflower seeds (1/4 cup) 18

Vitamin C (Mg.)

Red Pepper, raw (1/2 cup) 95
Honeydew (cup) 92
Papaya (cup) 87
Strawberries (cup) 84
Kiwi (med) 74
Orange (med) 70
Cantaloupe (cup) 68
Orange Juice (4 fl. oz.) 62
Product 19, Kellogg's (cup) 60
Total, General Mills (cup) 59
Mango (med) 57
Green Pepper (1/2 cup) 48
Cranberry Juice (4 oz) 45
Kohlrabi, cooked (1/2 cup) 45
Grapefruit, red/white (1/2 med) 43
Broccoli (1/2 cup) 39

Beta-Carotene (IU)

Carrot Juice (4 oz) 19
Sweet Potato, cooked (med) 17
Pumpkin, canned, cooked (1/2 cup) 16
Carrot, fresh, frozen, cooked (1/2 cup) 11
Mango (med) 5
Spinach, cooked (1/2 cup) 4
Cantaloupe (cup) 3
Apricot, dried (1/2 cup) 3
Winter Squash (1/2 cup) 3
Spinach, raw (cup) 3
Red Pepper, raw (1/2 cup) 2

Other Sources of Antioxidants

Flavones

Compound	Food Source
Apigenin	apple skins
Chysin	berries
Kaempferol	broccoli
Luteolin	celery
Rutin	cranberries
Sibelin	grapes
Quercetin	lettuce, olives, onions, parsley

Flavonones

Fisetin	citrus fruit
Hespiritin	citrus peel

Catechins

Catechin	red wine, tea, chocolate
Epigallocatechin	black tea, green tea, chocolate
Epigallocatechin gallante	green tea

Anthocyanins

Cyanidin	berries
Delphinidin	cherries

Malvidin	grapes and raspberries
Peonidin	red grapes
Petunidin	strawberries, tea, fruit peels

Step 3: Proper Rest

There have been studies documenting the relationships between sleep deprivation and immune system decrements. At least seven hours of sleep is recommended with more for individuals who already have compromised immune systems.

Step 4: Exercise

Regular exercise is important for immune system health, stress management, weight control, and disease prevention. This will be covered in detail in chapter 10 with very specific recommendations for everyone.

Step 5: Stress Management & Self Care

Stress management is crucial for a healthy immune system and disease prevention. Often times when people get sick—even with the common cold—they can connect it to being under a lot of stress.

There are now many books and research projects on the role of stress in disease. For example, the American Cancer Society is funding a study called "The stress and Immunity Partner Study." This project examines the physical and emotional well-being of the cancer patient's partner. Research shows that the partners of cancer patients report sleep and appetite disturbances, more frequent episodes of infections like the cold and flu, and worsening of their own medical conditions.

Dr. Bruce Rubin, in his book *Stress, Immune Function, & Health: The Connection* uses the latest research on humans and animals to discuss the effects of maternal stress on the offspring, how exercise affects immunity, and how emotions influence immune-related diseases.

Another book entitled *Cytokines, Stress, and Immunity* by Robert Good provides a comprehensive overview of how cytokines, which are polypeptides released by cells of the immune system to regulate other cells, play a large role in modulating the effects of the stress hormones, adrenaline and cortisol. This book, while geared toward researchers and clinicians, makes us realize that the functions of the immune system are largely controlled by cytokine-hormone interactions and the body's ability for cells to signal to one another, particularly in response to foreign substances.

Laughter should also be mentioned as part of building a healthy immune system. When I was sick I read the book *The Anatomy of an Illness*, by Norman Cousins. He was critically ill and relied on high doses of vitamin C and laughter to recover, much to the dismay of the medical community. The book had an impact on me, and since then I have read studies on the effects of laughter for pain management and disease prevention. I even attended a lecture given by a "Jolly-Ologist" who had us all practicing different types of laughs and truly enjoying the moment. I can't tell you how good I felt during the seminar and for hours afterwards. A good belly laugh can raise endorphins which can reduce pain and improve immune functioning. Endorphins are defined as neurotransmitters found in the brain with pain-relieving properties similar to morphine. Besides behaving as a pain regulator, endorphins are also thought to be connected to physiological processes including euphoric feelings, appetite modulation, and the release of sex hormones. So laugh often, and find pleasure in everyday activities.

Step 6: Nutritional Supplements

Nutritional supplements also boost the immune system. Many of these will be mentioned again in chapter 9. The focus here is on antioxidants to stop free radical damage.* I recommend a balanced multi-vitamin/mineral complex, natural vitamin E with mixed tocopherols,* selenium, vitamin C with bioflavanoids, mixed carotenoids and zinc. Glandular supplements like thymus* or adrenal* extracts and certain botanicals like echinacea, astragalus root, and garlic may be indicated for certain individuals on an as needed basis.

8

Eat to Boost Energy, Stay Fit and Maximize Health

After working with thousands of patients over the years, I have found the diet that generally works best is a balanced meal plan where approximately 40 % of the daily calories consumed are carbohydrates, 30 % protein, and 30 % fat. I favor this plan because it cuts down on carbohydrates consumed as in the popular Atkins and South Beach diets, but is less extreme and can therefore be followed for longer periods of time without consequences or major sacrifices.

The Dean Ornish heart healthy diet recommends 75% of the foods consumed should be carbohydrates, 15% protein and 10% fat. The current food pyramid suggests 60% of the diet should come from carbohydrates, 15% protein and 25% fat. The Atkins diet recommends 10% calories come from carbohydrates, 30% protein and 60% fat.

You can see why so many people are confused as to which food plans really work. The 40-30-30 plan is moderate. You don't have to cut out carbohydrates and as long as you consume the healthy ones (explained in detail later) you can have carbohydrates with each meal. There is also less fat than is recommended in the Atkins plan, and the fats recommended are the good fats, not the saturated kind. The protein amounts are the same.

Patients who do the Atkins or South Beach diets may lose weight faster than on the balanced 40-30-30 plan, but many gain the weight back once they start adding more grains and fruits. The 40-30-30 plan is also healthier overall and not as hard on the liver and kidneys.

The carbohydrates selected should be low glycemic and high fiber (see charts). The body needs to pump out a lot of insulin to process the foods high on the glycemic list. Low glycemic foods yield a slower rise in blood sugar and a more gradual release of insulin into the system. These foods are much better tolerated and will keep you more satisfied and less fatigued during the day as blood sugar stays steady. That's why when you have a plain bagel, white rice, or sugary cereal you are usually hungry and tired again in an hour. The foods that cause a rapid rise in blood sugar cause a quick fall, thus creating these symptoms. The more fiber these carbohydrates have the better, since fiber also slows down the blood sugar surge and insulin response. It also fills you up so you do not become hungry as quickly.

The glycemic Index is a system that rates how fast certain foods increase blood sugar levels and how quickly the body responds by bringing levels back to normal. Research indicates faster fat loss using low or medium glycemic index carbohydrates. Foods with a lower glycemic index usually contain more protein, fat, and fiber.

GLYCEMIC INDEX

This chart will help you select foods that will keep your blood sugar under control and keep you burning body fat.

Selected Glycemic Foods Ranked Low, Medium, and High

Fruit—Generally low, dried fruits, mangos, cantaloupe, papayas, and bananas are medium.

Vegetables—Generally low, beets and corn are medium, and white potatoes are high.

Cereals—All Bran, Kashi, oatmeal, and Special K are low. Grape Nuts are medium. Bran flakes, Raisin Bran, Cheerios, and Corn Flakes are high.

Bread—Most breads are high except for Eziekel and 100% Stone Ground Whole wheat.

Pasta—Most pasta is medium, whole wheat pasta is low.

Other Grains—White rice, millet, and rice cakes are high. Brown and basmati rice are medium. Barley and oats are low.

Junk Foods—Pretzels, chips, candy, and crackers are all high. Ice Cream is medium due to the high level of fat and some protein.

Protein Foods—Meat, fish, poultry, eggs, soy, and nuts are low.

Beans—Black eyed peas, butter beans, chickpeas, lentils, lima beans, navy, pinto are low. Baked beans are medium.

Dairy Products—Milk and cheese are low.

Sugars—All sugars, honey, maple syrup, maltose are high.

The average American consumes 10-15 grams of fiber per day. In order to achieve the maximum heart protection and to prevent diabetes it is recommended that 25-35 grams of fiber a day should be consumed. Not only does this help with weight reduction, but it also helps with cholesterol management and digestive health, as fiber cleanses the colon and helps the body's natural detoxification process. One caveat to adding too much fiber to the diet at once is that it could cause gas in some individuals. Another is that if you add more fiber to the diet without adding enough fluid to balance it out it could cause constipation as there is not enough liquid to push the fiber through the colon. Add fiber slowly and drink 64 ounces of water a day for maximum benefit.

THE HIGH-FIBER DIET

Food	Fiber Content (grams)
Bread	
French	0.7/1 slice
Rye	0.8/1 slice
White	0.7/1 slice
Whole wheat	1.3/1 slice

Cereal

Kashi Go Lean	10/1 cup
All Bran (100%)	8.4/1/3 cup
Corn Flakes	2.6/3/4 Cup
Wheaties	2.6/3/4 cup
Shredded Wheat	2.8/1 biscuit

Crackers/Snacks

Graham	1.4/2 squares
Rye	2.3/3 wafers
Saltine	0.8/6 crackers
Popcorn	3.0/3 cups

Vegetables

Asparagus	3.5/1/2 cup
Bean sprouts	1.5/1/2 cup
Broccoli	3.5/1/2 cup
Brussels sprouts	2.3/1/2 cup
Cabbage	2.1/1/2 cup
Carrots, raw	1.8/1/2 cup
Cauliflower	1.6/1/2 cup
Celery, raw	1.1/1/2 cup
Corn	2.6/1/2 ear
Eggplant, raw	2.5/1/2 cup
Kale greens	1.3/1/2 cup
Lettuce	.8/1 cup
Onions, raw	1.2/1/2 cup

Peas, canned	6.7/1/2 cup
Potatoes	
White, baked	1.9/1/2 medium
Sweet	2.1/1/2 medium

Beans

Navy	8.4/1/2 cup
Kidney	9.7/1/2 cup
Lima	8.3/1/2 cup
Pinto	8.9/1/2 cup
String	2.1/1/2 cup

Fruit

Apple	2.0/1/2 large
Apricots	1.4/2
Banana	1.5/1/2 medium
Blackberries	6.7/3/4 cup
Cherries	1.1/10 large
Grapefruit	0.8/1/2 grapefruit
Grapes, white	0.5/10 grapes
Orange	1.6/1 small
Peach	2.3/1 medium
Pear	2.0/1/2 medium
Pineapple	0.8/1/2 cup
Plums	1.8/3 small
Raspberries	9.2/1 cup
Strawberries	3.1/1 cup

Besides starches, fruits and vegetables also come under the carbohydrate category. I usually advise my weight-loss and Syndrome X risk patients to fill up on vegetables. Five to nine servings a day is ideal, and one should also have two to three whole fruits a day. The starch recommendation is individual depending on the goals of the patient, but usually three to five servings are recommended for slow steady weight loss depending on the size of the person and how quickly they want to lose weight. The following chart will show you what a serving size consists of. You will see that it is easy to get a serving of vegetables, and a serving of starch is a lot smaller than you think.

Basic Serving Sizes for Common Foods

Fruits: 1/2 banana, grapefruit, mango, papaya; one apple, kiwi, nectarine, peach, pear; two small plums, ten grapes; 1/2 cup unsweetened pineapple, 3/4 cup blueberries, two dates or medium prunes.

Fats

one Tbsp. flaxseed, pumpkin seed or walnut oil
one Tbsp. extra virgin olive, peanut, high-oleic safflower, or sunflower oil
one Tbsp. pine nuts or sunflower seeds
1/4 cup almonds, walnuts, cashews
1/8 medium avocado

Vegetables

1/2 cup cooked vegetables or raw salad greens such as broccoli, eggplant, red and green peppers, lettuce, spinach, zucchini, watercress, cauliflower, one stalk celery, one tomato, one carrot or six baby carrots

Protein

Four oz. tofu or tempeh, two eggs, four oz. fatty fish or shellfish, four oz. cooked meat, poultry, lamb, veal

Starches

one cup cooked barley, basmati, or brown rice
one cup dried black, garbanzo, kidney, navy, pinto, soy beans
1/2 cup corn or winter squash
3/4 cup peas or pumpkin
1/2 whole grain bagel
one small pita pocket or slice of bread
3/4-one cup most cereals

Dairy

one oz. farmer, goat, string, most hard cheeses
four oz. skim ricotta or low-fat cottage cheese
six oz. plain nonfat or low-fat yogurt
eight oz. goats milk, nonfat cows milk

The protein selected should be high quality and low-fat, such as poultry without the skin, fish, soy, beans, and egg whites, and for some people low-fat dairy, and certain cuts of meat. All products are best if they can be certified organic and minimally processed, in particular hormone and antibiotic free. The reason why I put red meat and dairy separately is that these foods are high in arachidonic acid* which can cause inflammation in the body. If someone has an auto-immune disease, arthritis or other pro-inflammatory condition it is best if they use a minimum amount of these foods. Also there is concern that many people have dairy intolerances. I have seen many of my patients with migraines, asthma, reflux, psoriasis, and other allergic types of conditions improve significantly when dairy products are reduced or eliminated. Some patients who have heart disease are told to eliminate red meat and eggs from their diet. Frequently eating foods like prime rib, other fatty cuts of meats, bacon, and eggs can be troublesome for many, but having three egg yolks a week with unlimited amount of whites, and eating lower-fat, grain fed meat like flank steak can be nutritious. Red meat remains one of the best sources of iron and zinc, and many menstruating women feel that it gives them more energy than they can get from plant foods. I recommend organic, grain or grass fed meat to eliminate any problems from excess hormones or antibiotics in the animal feed.

The last category is fats. Like carbohydrates and protein, this area is totally dependent on the kind of fats chosen.

Most of us think about what fat does to our waistlines; however, the right kind of fat can help with weight balance and hormonal health, prevent heart disease and assist neurotransmitters to the brain which prevent depression, mood swings, memory loss, and attention/focus problems. In addition, fat, like fiber and protein, is digested slowly in the body and gives us a sense of fullness after a meal. When the fat component is approximately 30% of the meal, there is a better chance that you will not be hungry again for three to four hours, when it may be time to eat a healthy balanced snack.

The following are recommended fats and the ones to use sparingly:

Recommended Fats

- According to the American Heart Association, mono-unsaturated fats found in almond, canola, olive and peanut oils and poly-unsaturated fats found in corn, soybean, safflower and sunflower oils may have cholesterol-lowering effects when used in place of saturated fats in the diet. Polyunsaturated fatty acids tend to help the body get rid of newly formed cholesterol. They keep the blood cholesterol level down and reduce cholesterol deposits in the artery walls. Monounsaturated fatty acids may also help reduce blood cholesterol when the diet is low in saturated fat without lowering HDL, the good cholesterol.

- Essential fats are the fats that we need to get from our diet because our bodies cannot manufacture their own. Examples are omega-3 fats found in fish oils, plant algae, and flax. The highest amounts of these oils are found in wild salmon, sardines, mackerel, and fresh tuna. Due to the high mercury content in tuna and farm raised salmon I would limit consumption of these fish to no more than once a month. The other essential fats are omega-6 fats found in nuts, seeds, and evening primrose or borage seed oils. Essential fats are converted into prostaglandins,* which are critical to the regulation of our entire physical system—from growth and tissue repair to energy production and fat metabolism.

Eliminate or Use Rarely

- Saturated fats are found in palm and coconut oils, cocoa butter, and in high fat meats and dairy products. The foods with the highest amounts of saturated fatty acids are beef and beef products, poultry skin, lard, butter, cream, whole milk and cheeses, and other dairy products. They also contain dietary cholesterol.

- Trans-fats are found in hydrogenated and partially hydrogenated oils. These are altered fats thought to be worse than saturated fats on blood lipid levels and could possibly cause cancer if consumed in large quantities. They are used to prolong the shelf-life of snack foods like crackers and cookies. According to an article by Dr. Bruce Fife, a certified nutritionist and naturopathic physician, recent research shows that trans-fats are far more dangerous than any other fat known. He points to a study published in the *American Journal of Clinical Nutrition* which reported that trans-fatty acids cause at least 30,000 premature deaths in the United States each year. In his article he states "because of these dangers, many health organizations have pressured the FDA to enact a regulation requiring food manufactures to include the amount of trans fatty acids on package labels. The FDA waited three years for the Institute of Medicine to study the issue. After a detailed review, the Institute of Medicine released their findings. They announced that no level of trans fat is safe to consume."

- Fried foods are cooked at such high temperatures that the vegetable oil usually used is turned to trans-fats and therefore equally
unhealthy.

I find the best daily meal plan for most people to start with, consists
of 3 balanced meals using the 40-30-30 philosophy just explained and
two balanced snacks. If you were going to follow a 1500-1800 calorie a
day meal plan (good for an inactive person who weighs between 130-
160 lbs.) then the calories should be roughly 400-500 per meal and
about 100-200 per snack. If you are active or weigh between 170-200
lbs. the daily requirements are approximately 2,000-2,500 calories and
could be broken down to 600 calories per meal and several snacks during the day. If you weigh less than 130 your caloric requirements are
between 1200-1500 calories a day.

Dietary recommendations are often confusing. Here is an example
of a balanced meal plan that is high in antioxidants, essential fatty
acids, fiber, and quality protein that uses the basic 40-30-30 principles.
Pick the meal and snack choices that most appeal to you and feel free
to substitute fruit, vegetable, and protein choices.

I recommend that you choose three meals and two snacks from the
following list. This works well for weight management, blood sugar
balance and improved focus and attention.

Breakfast Choices

One cup oatmeal, six oz. organic, low fat milk or soymilk, two tbsp.
fresh ground flax meal, 1 scoop protein powder

or

Two oz. smoked salmon, one tbsp. reduced-fat organic cream cheese or
soft goat cheese, small whole wheat pita pocket

or

Two soft boiled or poached eggs, one slice whole grain toast, green tea

or

One cup hot brown rice cereal, ½ banana, ¼ cup almonds or walnuts

or

Eight oz. no-fat plain yogurt, one cup strawberries, one tbsp. flax oil, ¼ cup nuts

or

¾ cup organic cottage cheese, one tbsp flax oil, ¾ cup blueberries

or

One whole grain bran muffin, one tbsp. almond butter or natural peanut butter, six oz. organic milk or soymilk

or

Egg white omelette with mushrooms, green pepper, and onions, one oz. goat cheese, one slice whole grain toast or fruit

or

Protein shake with two scoops protein powder, organic milk, soymilk, or yogurt, and one fruit

or

One cup high fiber, low sugar cereal such as Kashi, All-Bran, or Grape-Nuts with ¼ cup nuts, organic skim milk, soymilk or goat milk

or

Whole grain waffle with soy and flax meal, fresh berries, a dribble of syrup or all-fruit jam

or

Three-four Ryvetta crackers with goat cheese and cut up strawberries on top

or

Breakfast parfait with four oz. yogurt, ½ cup high fiber cereal, and ½ cup strawberries; add in your favorite protein powder

Lunch & Dinner Choices

Four slices white turkey meat, Dijon mustard on Ezekiel* bread or small pita, spinach salad with flax & olive oil dressing

or

Four oz. crabmeat, one tbsp. low-fat mayonnaise, chopped celery, romaine lettuce, tomato, one slice whole grain bread, side mixed green salad

or

Stir fried tofu with snow peas, onion, bean sprouts, red pepper over ½ cup brown rice

or

Two Bean burritos with green salad with flax & olive oil vinaigrette

or

Mixed grilled veggie wrap with side spinach salad with olive oil & vinegar dressing

or

Seasoned sardines in water with mixed green salad and dressing choice

or

Four oz. broiled red snapper, steamed broccoli, baked yams

or

Large mixed green salad with oil and lemon juice, four oz. free range chicken on top with chopped yellow and sweet red peppers

or

Four oz. stuffed flounder wrapped with spinach and low-fat feta cheese over ½ cup brown rice mixed with carrots and zucchini

or

Lentil and brown rice casserole with mixed vegetables and two oz. goat cheese

or

Chicken salad sandwich made with free-range chicken, low-fat canola mayonnaise on high fiber bread with lettuce and tomato and roasted vegetables

or

Soy or free-range turkey, buffalo, or venison burger on whole wheat bun with lettuce, tomato, and onion, and veggie slaw on the side

or

Quinoa* bean salad with chopped celery, onion, carrots, zucchini, and white beans over romaine lettuce

or

Mixed green salad with one oz. goat cheese, cut up pear, ¼ cup wal-nuts, and poppy seed dressing

or

Brown rice stir fry with vegetable medley and black beans seasoned with soy sauce or Bragg's amino acid dressing

Snacks

Almond or natural peanut butter on apple or celery

or

Protein shake with freshly ground flax seeds

or

¼ cup of nuts with one fruit

or

Eight small whole grain crackers with one oz. low-fat cheese

or

One serving soy chips or baked lays with salsa

or

Hard boiled egg

or

Two oz. lean hormone-free turkey, ham or cheese rolled with mustard

or

Balanced protein bar without corn syrup or hydrogenated oil

or

Guacamole and one serving baked chips

or

One serving baked chips with hummus

Beverages

Purified Water
Seltzer plain or flavored
Organic skim milk, soymilk or goat milk
Green tea
Herbal non-caffeinated tea
De-caffeinated coffee or tea
Green drinks—high in chlorophyll,* which helps keep the system alkaline*
Fresh mixed vegetable juice (low in carrot and beet which are high in sugar)

I hope that many of the meal suggestions appeal to you using the balanced diet approach. If you feel that it is an extreme change from what you are used to I recommend that you start slowly. For instance you may start by cutting down on sugar, alcohol or caffeine initially and when you feel you can take on another challenge add one more change. Most people report more energy, better sleep, and less irritability when they work on these three big changes. Some of my patients report better skin, hair, and digestion, especially when they have been constipated, just by upping their water intake to 64 oz/day. Everybody is different. Find your own balance of what you can give up based on your health goals and level of commitment.

There is a rule that many nutritionists share with their clients who are just beginning the diet make over process. That is the 80-20 rule. If you follow my recommendations 80% of the time, then 20% of the time you can eat what you want without guilt. Have an occasional glass of wine or dessert at dinner. Have an ice cream, burger or fries now and then. It's when we deprive ourselves all of the time that we tend to feel cheated and that's when many of us abandon the healthy eating plan altogether and revert to old eating habits. When we recognize that no food is 100% forbidden and we can have our treats on occasion, the program becomes more livable in the long-term.

On that note, I want to talk to you about a food that many of my patients have trouble giving up: chocolate. There is something so seductive and irresistible about chocolate, especially for those of you with PMS. The good news is that this is one food you could use occasionally and feel good about it, because it is good for you. Chocolate has many health benefits—that is, if you consume the dark chocolate with high cocoa content. This type of chocolate has a high flavanoid content, is an anti-oxidant, and according to in vitro observations has been shown to have an anti-cancer effect similar to certain fruits and vegetables. It is also high in the minerals potassium, iron, magnesium, zinc, and copper. According to the latest research, milk (as in milk chocolate) may decrease the absorption of the dietary flavanols and thus minimize the healing effects.

The downside to chocolate is its high calories. One medium bar of dark chocolate has about 210 calories and at least 13 grams of fat. It could also cause problems for people who have gastric reflux and are prone to migraines and food allergies. So use it sparingly, but when you indulge, lose the guilt.

If you find that you follow my dietary, exercise and stress management recommendations 80% of the time, but are still not feeling well and not losing weight, then you most likely have some imbalances that need to be corrected. Many of these—thyroid functioning, hormone or mineral imbalances, and food sensitivities—were discussed in previous chapters. There are also a growing number of nutritionists like myself who are using metabolic typing to help people who cannot improve regardless of the nutritional or other programs they try. Metabolic typing is based on the concept of biochemical individuality. We all have come from different ancestors and have different metabolic chemistries, so our needs for foods and supplements are varied. In his book, *The Metabolic Typing Diet,* William Wolcott speaks of his process of metabolic typing which involves the evaluation of the interrelationships among the autonomic nervous system, the oxidative system, and seven additional physiological parameters that influence body chemistry.

Lastly I want to cover the subject of eating out. Many of my patients report staying on their sensible food plans during the week only to gain weight on the week-end after over indulging at their favorite restaurants. If you eat out infrequently then follow the 80/20 rule previously mentioned. Some of my patients eat out almost all of their meals. That is when you have to be super careful and make sure you follow these simple guidelines:

1. Don't go to a restaurant starving. Have a glass of water with fiber mixed in or a handful of nuts to fill you up before you go.

2. Ask the waiter to leave the bread off the table. If you have a small piece of bread dip it in olive oil so that the fat of the oil will slow down the glycemic response of the bread. Fat will also give you a sense of fullness, whereas the bread alone will increase your hunger.

3. Order a green salad with dressing on the side, cut up vegetables or a clear soup (non-creamy) as an appetizer.

4. For your main meal order lean protein such as chicken, turkey, or fish and have a double serving of vegetables instead of rice, potato, or pasta. If the serving is to large, segment half of the meal apart and have that wrapped up to take home.

5. The protein consumed should be baked, roasted, broiled, grilled or boiled, not fried or made with cheese or other cream sauces.

6. For beverage choose water or sparkling water with lemon or lime. An occasional glass of wine is okay.

7. For dessert the best choices are fresh fruit, or non-fat frozen yogurt.

8. Don't be intimidated to choose right off of the menu! Make sure to order the food that you want cooked the way you like it.

9

Vital Herbs and Nutritional Supplements: A Three Phased Program

Throughout the pages of this book I have recommended nutritional supplements that help a variety of conditions. Those of you who are in general good health and eat a balanced, varied diet don't need to take a host of supplements. If you follow the recommended better health diet you will be getting a good ration of protein, carbohydrates and healthy fat as well as vitamins, minerals, and fiber.

Many people don't like to take a lot of pills, but it's hard to get everything from diet alone. Fruits and vegetables are grown in soil that is largely mineral deficient. Choosing certified organic fruits and vegetables will provide more nutrients. However, before we eat our food it is early harvested, shipped and stored, all of which depletes the nutrient content. Therefore, even those with a well balanced diet should consider some basic supplements.

The three phase supplement plan that follows offers something for everyone. Use the first phase if you are healthy, have good genes, follow a good diet and dislike taking a lot of pills. Use the second phase if you have a lot of stress in your life but otherwise are in good health. Use the third phase if you want to focus more on prevention and longevity. Supplements in the third phase are more important as we age and our bodies slow down or stop working the way they once did.

Phase I—The Must Haves Supplements for Everyone

1. Multi-vitamin and mineral complex with at least:

- 400 mcg. of Folic Acid—Prevents birth defects, helps with heart health.

- 400 I.U. of Vitamin D—Important for bone health, growth, and calcium absorption.

- 15 mg. of Zinc—Important for immune and skin health, memory and concentration, and blood sugar balance.

- 300 mcg. of Biotin—Important for hair health and blood sugar balance.

- 450 mg. of Calcium—Important for bone and colon health, natural muscle relaxer.

- 200 mg. of Magnesium—Important for calcium absorption, heart health, and blood sugar balance. Also natural muscle relaxer.

- 100 mcg. of Selenium—Anti-oxidant, helps detoxify the body.

- 100 mcg. of Chromium—Important for blood sugar balance and insulin metabolism.

Most multi-vitamins do not have enough of the following nutrients. I therefore recommend that you take these in addition to your multi:

2. 400 I.U. of natural Vitamin E with mixed tocopherols—For heart disease prevention, and hormonal, neurological, and immune health. For those of you concerned about the November 10, 2004 article in the online issue of *Annals of Internal Medicine* which stated that vitamin E increased mortality rates, rest assured that this data was sensationalized by the media based on individuals who had existing conditions such as cancer, heart disease, Alzhe-

imer's, Parkinson's and kidney failure. In addition, the study did not differentiate between natural and synthetic vitamin E and used just alpha tocopherol instead of the mixed kind which is what is found in food. Many positive studies have recognized vitamin E's protective qualities on the general population and several publications have come out with rebuttals to this study recommending Vitamin E up to 1600 I.U.'s for normal, healthy adults.

3. 500 mg. of Vitamin C—Good for immune health, and healthy skin and gums.

4. Omega-3 supplement (1,000-2,000 mg.)—If you do not get at least one tbsp. a day of flax oil or eat fish highest in Omega-3 oils (wild salmon, sardines, mackerel, fresh tuna) on a regular basis.

5. Calcium 1000 mg./Magnesium 500 total intake for the day—This is what most people need. Women who are pregnant, teens, and people with osteoporosis have greater needs. It is best to see what you get from your diet and multi-vitamin and balance the rest with an additional supplement if necessary. I think it is important to have close to a two to one ratio when picking a calcium and magnesium supplement. There should be two parts calcium to one part magnesium, unless you have a tendency toward constipation or diarrhea. A ratio of one part calcium to one part magnesium is better if you are prone towards constipation as calcium can be binding and worsen your symptoms. If on the other hand you are prone to loose stools then three to one calcium to magnesium ration may be best, since magnesium can cause loose stools. Magnesium and vitamin D are crucial for calcium absorption. Choosing a supplement that has all three together generally works best.

Here are some common sources of dietary calcium:

- 1 cup of milk, fat-free or 1%—300-350 mg.
- 1 cup of soymilk, fortified—200-400 mg.

- 1 cup of Yogurt, fat-free or low-fat, plain—350-400 mg.
- 1 cup of Fortified orange juice—350 mg.
- 1/2 cup of Tofu—200 mg.
- 1 cup of Cottage cheese, low-fat—140 mg.
- 1 cup of Sardines canned in water, drained—320 mg.
- 1 oz. of Swiss cheese—220 mg.
- 1 oz. of Cheddar cheese—200 mg.
- 1/2 cup of Ricotta cheese—200 mg.
- 1 cup of Bok choy—200 mg.
- 1 cup of Kale—200 mg.
- 1 cup of Broccoli—80 mg.
- 1 cup of Turnip greens—200 mg.
- 1/2 cup of Canned salmon, including bones—200 mg.
- 1/2 cup of Ice Cream or frozen yogurt, low-fat or fat-free—75-150 mg.

Here are some of the best sources of dietary magnesium:

- 1 cup of Spinach, cooked—160 mg.
- 1 cup of Oysters, raw—130 mg.
- 1/4 cup of Sesame seeds, dry—120 mg.
- 1/2 cup of Tofu—115 mg.
- 1 cup of Beet Greens, cooked—100 mg.
- 1 cup of Garbanzo beans, cooked—75 mg.
- 3 oz. of Sole/flounder, baked—50 mg.
- 1 cup of Yogurt, nonfat—50 mg.
- 1 cup of Milk, nonfat—25 mg.

Phase II Supplements—For Those with Increased Stress
Follow Previous Program and Add:

1. B-Complex—Found primarily in whole grain and enriched bread products, dairy, meat, and leafy green vegetables. Find a B-supplement that contains all 8 components of the B family in proper balanced proportions.

2. Vitamin C—1500-2000 mg.—Found primarily in citrus fruits, cabbage, dark green vegetables, cantaloupe, strawberries, peppers, papayas, and mangoes.

Even though most multi-vitamins have the 8-B complex vitamins, they get burned up very quickly when under stress. In addition, the B vitamins help with blood sugar balance, reduce sugar cravings, and turn food into energy. Most of us experience some degree of stress. The B vitamins help manage stress better and create an overall sense of well-being.

Vitamin C also gets burned up very quickly when under stress. Since everyone's body is different, I recommend a range based on your life style and immune health. If you are a smoker you need the highest dose of vitamin C, since about 50 mg. of vitamin C is burned with each cigarette smoked. For everyone else, I recommend 1,000 mg. daily. Feel free to increase it to bowel tolerance if you feel an infection coming on or if you are doing a lot of traveling, are run down or preparing for surgery. Since vitamin C is water soluble, the body uses what it needs and gets rid of the rest. There is therefore no risk of storing too much as in the case of the fat soluble vitamins: A, E, and D.

Phase III Supplements—For Prevention and Longevity
Follow Previous Program and Add:

1. Coenzyme Q 10—A powerful antioxidant for energy and cellular function, particularly for the heart. This enzyme is especially important as we age and less is available to us naturally. Virtually every cell of the body contains CoQ10, but when we get older the body cannot synthesize it as well. It can be found in certain food sources like fish and meat but not in high enough quantities for therapeutic effect. The recommended dose is 30-100 mg. per day depending on the reason for usage. Many people go on statin drugs to lower their cholesterol levels. One of the reasons why these drugs work is that they close down a pathway in the body where cholesterol is manufactured. That same pathway is needed to produce CoQ10, making it even more important to take it if you are using these drugs.

2. I also suggest one or two supplements to help with brain function such as phosphatidylcholine,* a supplier of choline, which is needed for normal brain functioning or ginkgo biloba,* an herb that is widely used for memory and concentration by increasing blood flow to the brain. There have been limited studies that suggest both of these supplements could prevent Alzheimer's disease. More work needs to be done to prove or disprove these claims, but many of my patients have reported better memory, and improved focus and attention, when using these supplements. Since herbs act more like medicine than vitamins, check with your physician before adding ginkgo, especially if you are on blood thinners or other medication.

3. Based on the research previously cited, I recommend probiotics in powder or capsule form. Some companies now make good products that do not need to be refrigerated. I spoke about the impor-

tance of probiotics to some degree in the chapter on digestive health and in the children's health section. While many people take them to counteract the effects of antibiotics, they are also helpful to promote better digestion and absorption of nutrients. They provide gut level immune system protection, prevent yeast infections and bacterial overgrowth, counteract constipation, diarrhea, bloating, gas, and even inhibit H. pylori,* the common cause of ulcers and gastritis. A yogurt a day provides some protection. However, if you have digestive problems a yogurt does not provide enough quantity and variety of probiotic strains.

4. The last supplement that I want to mention is the herb Rhodiola Rosea. According to Richard Brown, MD and his wife Patricia Gerbarg, MD, the authors of the book *The Rhodiola Revolution,* this herb is scientifically proven to increase energy, fight the effects of stress and aging, sharpen memory and concentration, protect against heart disease and cancer, ease anxiety and depression, help balance hormones, improve sexual function, enhance physical performance, and block fat for lasting weight loss. If it does half of that it will truly be a miracle herb. I have been using Rhodiola with my patients over the last three months and have heard some wonderful reports, particularly to help with fatigue, stress and weight loss. There are few side effects or contraindications reported with Rhodiola.

10

Exercise to Improve Cardiovascular Conditioning, Strength and Flexibility

While I recommend some kind of an exercise program for all of my patients, their needs vary greatly by age, physical condition and goals. I therefore asked Mike Tadesco, co-owner of Body Fit Personal Training in Cross River, New York, to give his more detailed recommendations. Mike is an ACE certified Personal Trainer and a tri-athlete. Body Fit is a local fitness facility geared toward creating individualized programs for adults and teen-agers in a low-key, professional environment.

You might also seek advice from a personal trainer near you to help tailor a workout that suits your needs. This may be particularly important for those of you with injuries or other disabilities. Also, if you are on medication or have specific medical conditions please make sure that you have consent from your doctor before starting any new exercise program.

Body Fit Exercise Recommendations

1. Benefits of Exercise:

a. Optimum Fitness

Peak physical fitness is defined as the development of an optimal level of cardiovascular endurance, muscular strength, and flexibility, as well as the achievement and maintenance of ideal body weight. An individual must participate in cardiovascular, strength and flexibility exercise to achieve optimum physical fitness. Although everyone's individual needs vary, it is recommended that most people **at least** get the following weekly exercise: 30 minutes of cardiovascular exercise like walking, running, swimming, or dancing three times a week, 20-30 minutes of muscular conditioning like free weights, machines, or exercise bands, two to three times a week, and 15-30 minutes of flexibility training like yoga, pilates, or stretching, two to three times a week.

Since time to fit this in is often a problem for people, book your exercise routines into your calendar, work out with a friend to stay motivated, and reward yourself for a job well done (without food) after completing a successful week or two.

b. Cardiovascular Endurance

Cardiovascular, or cardio respiratory endurance, also referred to as aerobic fitness, describes the ability of the cardiovascular/cardio respiratory system (heart, lungs, blood vessels) to deliver an adequate supply of oxygen to exercising muscles. Blood must flow from the heart through blood vessels (vascular) to the lungs to pick up oxygen that can be delivered to exercising muscles. This is important for cardiovascular & immune health, stress management, and detoxification.

c. Muscular Strength

Muscular strength is the maximum amount of force a muscle or muscle group can develop during a single contraction. Muscular endurance is the number of repeated contractions a muscle or muscle group can perform against a resistance without fatiguing, or the length of time a contraction can be held without fatigue.

This helps you build overall body strength, improve posture, and prevent osteoporosis and injury.

d. Flexibility

Flexibility describes the amount of movement that can be accomplished at a joint (an articulation), such as the knee or shoulder, and is usually referred to as the "range of motion about a joint." Maintaining flexibility may help reduce the risk of injury, and can also help improve performance in many activities.

e. Body Composition

Body composition refers to the relative proportions of body weight in terms of lean body mass and body fat. Lean body mass represents the weight of water, muscle, bone and internal organs. Body fat represents the remaining fat tissue and is expressed as a percentage of total body weight. It is essential to maintain some body fat for normal physiological functions. For example, it serves as an insulator to conserve body heat, as metabolic fuel for the production of energy, and padding for protection. It is important to realize that you may be overeating even though you are not overweight. The key is to eat the right foods as defined earlier in chapter 8.

Waist to Hip Ratio (WHR)—The waist-to-hip ratio (the circumference of the waist divided by the circumference of the hips) is a simple method for determining body fat patterns. Ratios above 0.95 for men and 0.86 for women place the individual at significantly increased health risk for the diseases that were mentioned in chapter 2.

Weight Control & Exercise—When trying to lose weight, people eat less and exercise more than they normally do. When exercising, the body needs even more nutrients and protein than normal to maintain and build new muscle. To avoid muscle loss, eat a well balanced diet as recommended in chapter 8. I usually recommend that people eat a small amount of carbohydrates about 30-60 minutes before they work out. This will be easily burned as fuel. Then eat a meal with protein after the work-out to help with muscle recovery.

2. Different Training techniques

a. Cardiovascular Training

During exercise, more energy is needed to perform the activity. Because of this, the heart, lungs, and blood vessels have to deliver more oxygen to the cells to supply the required energy. When exercising for long periods, someone with a high level of cardio respiratory fitness is able to supply enough oxygen to the tissues with relative ease. The cardio respiratory system of a person with a low fitness level has to work much harder, therefore getting tired faster. This means a person that can supply and use more oxygen has a more efficient cardio respiratory system. As you exercise for a while you will see your cardio respiratory fitness level improve. Don't be discouraged if you cannot perform aerobic exercises for long periods of time when you first start. Ten to15 minutes may be all that you can handle in the beginning. As the exercise gets easier for you, slowly work up to the recommendations that follow.

i. Target Heart Rate Zone (THR)

1. This method of monitoring intensity of exercise calculates the exercise heart rate as a percentage of maximal heart rate. Maximal heart rate can be determined by a maximal functional capacity test, using a bicycle or treadmill ergometer, or by age predicted maximal heart rate tables, which frequently use the 220-age formula. For simplicity we will use the following method for estimating maximal heart rate:

Target Heart Rate = (220-age) x 60% to 90%

For example, to calculate a target heart rate for a 44-year old man, the following formula can be used:

220-44 = 176 (predicted max H.R.)

176 x 60% = 105.6 or 106

176 x 90% = 158.4 or 158

This individual's Target Heart Rate zone is 106-158.

From a physiologic point of view, this 60% to 90% range is the goal for cardio respiratory training benefits. Lower intensities, such as 50%-60%, are advised for beginners in the lower cardio respiratory fitness levels. Persons with very low fitness levels can benefit from training intensities as low as 40%. Exercise intensities as high a 75% to 90% may be more appropriate for those who are apparently healthy and in the higher fitness classifications. Overall, the average exercise intensity for healthy adults is usually between 65% and 75% of their max heart rate.

ii. Rate of Perceived Exertion

1. Exercise intensity also can be measured by assigning a numerical value (1 to 10) to subjective feelings of exercise exertion. The popular name for this method is the ratings of perceived exertion (RPE). RPE takes into account your perception of exercise fatigue, including psychological, musculoskeletal, and environmental factors. The RPE response also correlates very well with cardio respiratory and metabolic factors such as heart rate, breathing rate, oxygen consumption, and overall fatigue.

0	Nothing at all
0.5	Very, very weak
1	Very weak
2	Weak

3	Moderate
4	Somewhat strong
5	Strong
6	
7	Very strong
8	
9	
10	Very, very strong

Ratings of Perceived Exertion

iv. Other scales

1. There are other scales and other ways of gauging "ideal" levels of exertion, such as the ability to talk to someone while working out. If you are breathing so heavily that you can't carry on a conversation, then you might be working out too intensely. If you are practicing sprints or doing some other short term high aerobic activity this does not apply.

b. Muscular Strength Training

i. Muscular strength is very important to your overall health and fitness. Adequate levels of strength are necessary to perform your daily routines at home and work, without excessive fatigue or stress. Higher levels of muscular fitness also reduce the incidence of lower back pain and injury to the musculoskeletal system. Strong muscles also help your cardiovascular system in sustaining physical activity.

ii. Like all other organs and systems of the human body, muscles have to be taxed beyond their regular accustomed loads to increase in physical capacity. A combination of resistance, number of sets and frequency are involved in increasing strength.

c. Flexibility

iii. Flexibility is the ability to move a joint fluidly through its complete range of motion, for general health and physical fitness. Flexibility is reduced when muscles become short and tightened with disuse causing an increase in injury and strains. Those with greater flexibility may have a lower risk of future back injury.

FACT: Older adults with better joint flexibility may be able to drive an automobile more safely. (National Health Promotion and Disease Prevention Objectives, United States Department of Health and Human Services Public Health Services).

To maintain your flexibility and prevent injury, it is recommended that you participate in a stretching routine before and following exercise. To improve flexibility, it is recommended that you participate in an additional stretching routine or do yoga once a week.

3. Measuring Success

a. Girth Measurements

i. Girth measurements may be used alone or with skin fold measurements to assess body composition. While this method of assessment has been shown to be no more accurate than skin folds alone, it is valuable in evaluation of girth changes that result from resistance training and provides a good check of skin folds and other methods of assessment as body composition changes. The two primary sources of error in measuring girth are inconsistent tape placement during repeated measures, and variations in the tension placed on the tape during the measurement. You can minimize the first error by using the standardized sites described below. You can overcome the second error by using a cloth tape specifically designed for girth measurement. These tapes have a scale that standardizes the tension applied to the tape as each site is measured. Take the measurements at these sites:

1. Chest—at the nipple line during the midpoint of a normal breath

2. Waist—at the narrowest point, below the rib cage and just above the top of the hip bones

3. Hips—with feet together, at the level of the symphysis pubis in front, at the maximal protrusion of the buttocks in the back

4. Thigh—at the crotch level and just below the folds of the buttocks

5. Calf—at the maximal circumference

6. Ankle—at the minimal circumference, usually just above the ankle bone

7. Upper arm—at the maximal circumference; arm extended, palm up

8. Wrist—at the minimal circumference; arm extended, palm up

Record the measurements for comparison each time body composition is assessed.

b. BMI and Body Fat %

Body Mass Index and body fat % were mentioned earlier and should also be re-assessed as part of a program to measure your success. It is common when a person starts to do a lot of exercise that they won't lose weight but will lose inches and body fat instead, since muscle weighs more than fat. Many commercial scales now give these measurements in addition to weight. There are more accurate machines for measuring exact body fat percents that range in cost from hundreds to thousands of dollars. For most people the basic ones are fine and as accurate, within a couple of percentage points.

11

De-Stress to Quiet Your Mind and Calm Your Spirit

Infectious diseases are no longer the major cause of death in the United States. Instead we have heart disease and cancer, which are largely life style degenerative diseases with the body decaying from within. The good news is that we can prevent much of this through all of the methods previously mentioned and by practicing stress management techniques.

Although everyone experiences stress, not everyone handles it constructively. The body can and does routinely cope with short-term stress, whether it is physical or emotional. It is the chronic long term stress that causes the body to break down and leads to disease. Stress can be caused by little things such as being too hot or cold, or exposed to too much noise and travel, or bigger things like a death in the family, divorce, job change, injury, or illness. On the emotional side, fears, depression, anger, anxiety, and negative thoughts can all contribute to stress.

Many chemical changes take place in the body when we experience stress and a surge of the body's resources kick in to handle the "fight or flight" scenario. This starts a rapid flow of energy into the muscles, heart, and brain resulting from an increase in the production and release of the adrenal and stress hormones. Blood sugar rises, leading the pancreas to release increasing amounts of insulin; when chronic, this can cause insulin resistance and if uncontrolled, diabetes. Our heart and respiratory rates increase, causing increased blood pressure, and again, if chronic, can cause wear and tear on the heart. Muscles become tense, leading to symptoms like spasms, headaches, and backaches.

The immune system is challenged as well, resulting in a decrease in the white blood cell's ability to destroy germs. In part, this is due to the reduction in the production of interferon and other molecules of the immune system and depletion of nutrients like vitamins A, B, C, E, zinc and protein, all important for a strong defense.

Since the fight or flight reaction causes most of our blood and energy to go to the muscles, heart and brain, there are fewer reserves available for digestive and reproductive health. The body reduces its ability to naturally produce digestive enzymes so food is only partially digested, leading to bloating, gas, and indigestion. The colon is sluggish, causing constipation, diarrhea and ulcers as the protective lining of the gastrointestinal tract is compromised.

Stress can also affect reproductive health. Men experience prostate problems and impotency, and women experience worsening P.M.S., endometriosis, and impaired fertility.

Now that we covered many of the ways stress can influence the body and accelerate the disease process, below are ways to counteract the effects of stress.

There are four keys to reducing stress:

Step 1: Nutrition

Nutrition helps prevent and repair the damage stress does to the body. Eating foods rich in vitamins, minerals and protein will replace cells broken down by the stress response. This can be done with the balanced diet described before, using a rainbow diet with plenty of fresh, colorful fruits, vegetables, whole grains, and quality protein.

Avoid or reduce foods that compound stress the most. They are sugar, caffeine, white flour, and alcohol. A diet which is too high in animal protein, processed foods, and unhealthy fats can also exacerbate the effect of stress.

Drink plenty of water and eliminate regular use of diet soda, juice, and sports drinks like Gatorade which have about 60 grams of sugar per bottle.

Step 2: Identify Your Stressors

Once the nutrition and supplement programs that were discussed earlier are followed, the next step is to try to identify your stressors and make a plan to change them to de-stress. This can take a while and you might need the help of a qualified psychotherapist. There are also good books like *Coping With Stress—A Guide for Living* by James Williard Mills, Ph.D. which walks you through a process for identifying your stress and then learning to resolve conflicts, reduce demands and uncertainty, and complete unfinished business so that you can assume control again.

Step 3: Rest & Exercise

It is also important to ensure that you get plenty of rest (at least seven hours a night) and exercise at least 30-45 minutes three times a week (again, daily is ideal). If you have certain medical conditions this may be too much and even add more physical stress to your body. Make sure to check with your doctor if this is the case.

Step 4: Relaxation, Joy, & Laughter

I mentioned earlier that it is important to "go to your bliss station" every day and incorporate more joy and laughter into your everyday life. Give or get a hug, play a game, take a relaxing bath, go on a nature walk, play with your pets, tinker in the garden, watch a funny movie, listen to music, play an instrument, write in your journal, or read a book. Sometimes when I feel stressed I will go outside and see the sun shining through the trees or icicles glistening with a rainbow of colors. I feel invigorated. Suddenly my problems seem so much smaller as I look at the enormity of the world around me with all of its magnificence.

Other Healing Practices

There are many healing practices that can be effective tools in stress management. The following is a partial list. I recommend that you investigate and explore what feels right for you.

Massage

Reconnective healing, Reiki, and other energy or chakra balance work

Acupuncture

Yoga

Tai Chi or Chi Gong

Meditation

Visualization exercises

Deep breathing

Positive affirmations

Biofeedback

Journaling

Prayer

Cathy's Health Makeover—Stress Leading to Immune System Breakdown

Background

Cathy, a recent patient, came to see me because as she felt "wiped out," and could barely get out of bed and get to work. She continually had one bronchial infection after another, and couldn't get back her energy. The illness started after her husband lost his job and she was caring for an ailing parent.

Besides the immune system problems, Cathy was experiencing constipation, bloating, gas and chronic ringing in her ears. Her diet was better than most, but she lacked protein, especially for breakfast, and started the day with two cups of coffee. She also consumed a lot of dairy products, which is especially a problem with chronic upper respiratory infections.

Treatment

At the first visit I suggested Cathy eat more protein and cut down on milk and meat products consumed for three weeks. Both promote inflammation because of the high amount of arachidonic acid. I also suggested that she eat more fruits, vegetables, turkey, fish, and beans, and drink more water. I asked her to consider eliminating caffeine, alcohol, and sugar until she was 100 % better, as these strain the immune system. The supplements I recommended were a multi-vitamin and mineral complex, garlic, an immune boosting supplement with echinacea, black elderberry extract,* and zinc, and the herb astragalus. She was already taking vitamins E, C, B complex, and flax oil, which I encouraged her to continue.

Results

When Cathy came back for the first time, she said the cough was finally gone and she didn't miss eating so much dairy. During the second visit she actually said she was "jumping out of bed in the morning" refreshed with great energy for the whole day. There was no more ringing in the ears, she was thinking more clearly, and her aches and pains were gone.

Cathy attributed a lot of her success to giving up dairy, sugar, and caffeine. In addition, she felt that she had a better understanding and control of her stress and was able to say "no" in situations where she felt that doing one more thing would be too much for her. That is a good lesson for everyone to learn.

Cathy's Makeover: Before

Problem: Stress leading to immune system break down, gas, bloating, ringing in the ears	Cathy had repeated upper respiratory infections. She was weak, tired, and drained. Her problems began shortly after her husband lost his job and she was caring for an ailing parent.
Diet:	Cathy was very fond of cheese and ate several portions daily. She also consumed a fair amount of red meat and sugar.
Supplements:	Cathy took a generic brand of supplements that was not working for her. She took a daily multiple, B, C, and calcium.
Exercise:	Since she was sick so often, Cathy could barely get out of bed and had no energy for exercise.
Stress Mgt. & Self-Care:	When she first came in, Cathy was so busy worrying about everyone else's needs that she barely had time to think about herself. She knew she needed a break but didn't know how or what to do to help herself.

Cathy's Makeover: After Total Wellness Program

Problem: Stress leading to immune system breakdown, gas, bloating, ringing in the ears	Once she eliminated sugar and dairy products from her diet and took some of the suggested supplements to boost her immune system, Cathy recovered quickly. Her infections cleared up, energy improved, and most of her other symptoms subsided.
Diet:	Cathy followed my recommendation of completely eliminating dairy, red meat, caffeine, alcohol, and sugar for one month. After that she was able to add back these foods in small quantities without any problems. She added chicken, fish, beans, nuts, and fruits and vegetables with some healthy whole grains.
Supplements:	For a short time Cathy was on immune boosting supplements: garlic, echinacea, black elderberry extract, zinc, and the herb astragalus. These were discontinued once her infection cleared up. She also changed her daily vitamins to better quality ones.
Exercise:	Cathy began walking regularly and doing a weekly yoga class. She also did light weight training and strength and conditioning exercises that I gave her for home.
Stress Mgt. & Self-Care:	After she felt better, Cathy realized that she needed to de-stress. She found a way to cut back her work schedule and take some time for doing things she enjoyed every day. She wrote in a journal and learned to meditate as well.

Summary

1. There are over 1000 biochemical reactions that occur when we invoke the stress response.

2. Look at times in your life when you were sick. Usually you will find these were the times you had the most stress in your life.

3. Diet and supplements are key to managing and preventing distress on the body and associated diseases.

4. Everyone has individual needs. Work with a qualified psychologist or get a good book to help you define and re-frame your stress.

5. Work with qualified health care practitioners who specialize in using energy and body work to uncover blocked "chi," the body's life force or energy. Sometimes blocks can be traced back to early childhood traumas or illnesses that have made an imprint on our cellular memory, even though the trigger incidents are long forgotten.

6. Perform breath work via meditation, yoga, or tai chi to slow down the body and help you de-stress.

12

Conclusion

Book conclusions are difficult to write because you want to leave your reader with profound parting thoughts that haven't already been said. I pondered this notion for several days and then the answer hit me.

As I was writing the conclusion of this book, I woke up sick one morning, even though I follow everything in this book, every day, most of the time. My diet hadn't changed. I was still taking my supplements, but I had recently added to my stress load without taking proper precautions.

Even though writing this book was a wonderful experience, the extra work and time commitment on top of an already busy schedule added more physical and emotional stress to my life. The regular programs I followed for de-stressing were morning meditation and stretching, stating positive affirmations at bedtime, writing in my journal, playing the guitar, and walking my dog around our lake. Due to my commitments and ailing knee, I was missing many of these activities.

Once I realized this I had an "aha" moment and made a commitment to myself to get back to daily meditations, walks, writing in my journal, yoga and stretching and I started doing nightly tai chi exercises.

I might not be able to do all of these things every day, but I would do many of them during the course of the week, even if it meant getting the book out of the door a little bit later.

If I could take stock of my life, find out what was wrong, make the necessary changes and redefine them on an on-going basis, then so can you.

Good luck on your journey to Total Wellness and fulfillment. I know you can do it!

Glossary

Adaptive Herb—An herb that adapts to what the body needs in terms of treatment.

Adrenal Insufficiency or Adrenal Stress Burnout—A normal amount of stress is healthy and good. When someone is in a continual state of flight or fight stress, with little down time, it often leads to this unhealthy condition marked by fatigue, insomnia, and mental exhaustion.

Aloe leaf—Aloe leaf has been used to treat a variety of ailments since the earliest days of recorded history. It is often used today to give soothing comfort from burns to ulcers.

An alkaline system—Each food that we eat is either alkaline or acidic. Grains, protein and most fats are acidic and fruits and vegetables are alkaline. Keeping the system in balance is important for overall good health.

Anti-Oxidant—A substance that neutralizes harmful compounds called free radicals that are responsible for cellular damage.

Arachidonic Acid—An unsaturated fatty acid found in small amounts in human and most animal fats.

Astragalus—Considered an adaptive tonifying herb in Chinese medicine to support immunity and cardiovascular health.

Attention Deficit Hyperactivity Disorder (ADHD)—This is a mental disorder categorized by a persistent pattern of inattention and/or hyperactivity and impulsivity.

Autistic Spectrum Disorder (ASD)—Is a spectrum of mental disorders that can range from severe (no speech, eye contact, or social interactions) to mild where there is speech, eye contact and some social ability.

Bioflavanoids—A live compound found in the pits, rinds, and seeds of citrus fruits and some other plants.

Black Elderberry Extract—Used to treat colds and bronchial infections.

Boswellia—An Ayurvedic herb that is used in the treatment of respiratory, digestive, and inflammatory diseases.

Bromelain—A plant enzyme extracted from pineapple, used to help in the digestion of proteins, reduce blood clotting, counter inflammation, and boost immunity.

Carotenoids—Organic chemical compounds naturally occurring in several forms in plants and producing an orange or red color. Examples of foods high in carotenoids are carrots and sweet potatoes.

Chasteberry Extract or Vitex—This adaptive herb is used for female hormone problems such as PMS, perimenopause, and infertility.

Chlorophyll—Comes from green foods. Helps keep the system alkaline. Chlorella and alfalfa are examples of nutrient sources that are high in chlorophyll.

Choline—A compound found in animal tissue as lecithin and acetylcholine which helps to prevent fat from being deposited in the liver.

Colitis—Inflammation of the colon, which may be acute or chronic. Often there are lower-bowel spasms, loose stools, and abdominal cramps.

Copper Toxicity—Indication of a high level of copper relative to zinc and other minerals that can be detected from a hair analysis.

CoQ10—An enzyme found naturally in the body in small quantities. It is used as a nutritional supplement primarily to improve heart health and boost energy.

Crohn's Disease—A chronic inflammatory disease, usually of the lower intestinal tract, marked by scarring and thickening of the intestinal wall.

Cysteine—A sulfur containing amino acid that is converted to cystine during metabolism.

Dandelion Root—Helps the body eliminate unwanted toxins. Works with milk thistle to reverse liver damage.

Deglycyrrhizinated Licorice (DGL)—Licorice root that is used to help with digestive problems such as ulcers and gastric reflux. The deglycyrrhizinted form does not cause a rise in blood pressure like regular licorice root.

Echinacea—A family of wildflowers known as the purple coneflower that has become a natural remedy for the common cold and flu.

EPA/DHA—Omega—3 fatty acids found in fish or fish oils.

Epstein Barr Virus (EBV)—This is the same virus that causes mononucleosis. Epstein Barr Virus or EBV is one of several common viruses that may be associated with Chronic Fatigue Syndrome. The symptoms are usually sore throat, swollen glands, foggy brain, and debilitating fatigue.

Epstein Barr Virus titers—The titers are used to measure the virus in blood serum. An Epstein Barr Virus titer test can test for old or current, active infection. Once you have this virus the titers will always be positive for old infection.

Ezekiel Bread—A sprouted multi-grain bread that is high in fiber and has a low glycemic index.

Fiber—The Coarse fibrous substances in grains, fruits, and vegetables that aid digestion and cleanse the intestines. Also called dietary fiber.

Follicle Stimulating Hormone (FSH)—A hormone that stimulates the growth of egg follicles in the ovaries.

Free Radical Damage—When the body is damaged by highly reactive and unstable molecules, usually associated with cell damage and aging.

Gastric Reflux—A condition which occurs when stomach acid comes up the digestive tract and causes symptoms such as heartburn, coughing and belching.

Ginkgo Biloba—An herb that is used primarily to improve memory and other mental functions. It is also used for vascular problems and tinnitus.

Glucosamine Sulfate—A dietary supplement used by the body to repair damage to joints caused by osteoarthritis or injury.

Glucose Regulation Complex—A supplement designed to improve glucose metabolism for those who have trouble regulating blood sugar or who are diabetic or pre-diabetic. This supplement contains the following ingredients: chromium, vanadium, magnesium, alpha lipoic acid, and taurine. There is more information about it in the reference section.

Glutamine—An amino acid that supports gastrointestinal mucosal healing.

Glutathione—A powerful anti-oxidant (see anti-oxidant) that is particularly helpful in the body's natural detoxification process.

Glycemic Index—This scale or index was originally designed for diabetics to let them know how quickly carbohydrates turn to sugar in the body. Glucose or table sugar has the highest glycemic index of 100. All foods on the list are measured against that baseline.

H. pylori—A common bacteria thought to be the main cause of ulcers and gastritis.

High Prolactin—Prolactin is a hormone secreted by the pituitary gland that stimulates lactation and the secretion of progesterone. High prolactin is sometimes a cause of infertility.

Homocysteine—An amino acid derived from proteins in the diet that can build up in the blood and contribute to the development of heart disease. Blood levels can now be easily detected to see if this is a problem. The remedy is to supplement with vitamins: B6, B12, and folate.

In Vitro Fertilization (IVF)—A procedure by which the sperm and eggs are fertilized in a laboratory and then implanted to increase chances of pregnancy.

Interstitial Cystitis—A chronic bladder disease that is caused by inflammation of the bladder wall.

Irritable Bowel Syndrome—A catch all diagnosis when a patient has frequent gastrointestinal pain, which may come with either constipation or diarrhea or vary between the two and no other diagnosis can be made.

Iso-flavones—The beneficial ingredient in soy and other plant products that helps with symptoms such as hot flashes and may be a factor in preventing heart disease.

Laparotomy—This is a surgical procedure where an incision is made along the abdomen area along the bikini line to remove a cyst or other growth.

L-Carnitine—An amino acid that can significantly increase fatty acid oxidation in adults. L-Carnitine is needed to transport fats from storage to be utilized.

L-Tyrosine—An amino acid that is the precursor of epinephrine, thyroxin, and other hormones.

Luteal Phase Defect—A condition that occurs in a women's cycle when there is not enough progesterone in the mid-cycle after ovulation to sustain a pregnancy.

Marshmallow Root—This herb is made from a sticky substance which makes it effective as a cough suppressant, would healer, and treatment for digestive problems such as crohn's and colitis.

Meridians—Refers to energy points along the body. Some alternative practitioners use meridian testing to see if the body's energy centers are in balance.

Methionine—A sulfur containing amino acid that occurs in proteins or can be prepared synthetically.

Milk Thistle (Silymarin)—One of the oldest herbal medicines used to help with liver problems.

Mixed Tocopherols—Natural antioxidants with biological activity found in vegetable oils. They occur in four derivatives: alpha, beta, gamma, and delta. The alpha form is commonly known as vitamin E.

MSM—Methylsulfonylmethane is an organic sulfur containing compound that occurs naturally in a variety of fruits, vegetables, grains, and animal products. The supplement form is used primarily to aid in pain management and for detoxification.

Pervasive Developmental Disorder (PDD)—A mild form of autism where there are developmental delays but the individual is much higher functioning then someone who is autistic.

Probiotic—Live beneficial bacteria that help increase resistance to pathogens such as salmonella and candida, and stimulate the immune system.

Prostaglandins—Precursors to hormones that occur naturally in all mammals.

Quercetin—This compound is found in the rind and bark of many plants and is used to treat a variety of conditions from abnormally fragile capillaries to sinus and allergy problems.

Quinoa—A high protein grain that can be substituted for wheat or rice in the diet. It cooks in about 15 minutes and is a low-fat source of dietary fiber and a complete protein.

Saccharomyces Boulardi—This is a safe and effective type of micro flora that helps to maintain intestinal health and normal bowel function. It is especially helpful to reduce the number of stools and to improve stool consistency.

Sensory Integration Dysfunction (SID)—Refers to people who have trouble processing sensory information. The symptoms are varied and can include being sensitive to sounds, touch and other stimulation or having problems with the taste or texture of food.

Slippery Elm—Slippery Elm made from tree bark is an herb that has been used for digestive health, sore throats, and even bad breath.

Taurine—A derivative of cysteine found in the bile, nervous tissue, and muscle juices of many animals.

Thymus or Adrenal Extracts—The thymus is an organ located at the base of the neck that is involved in cellular immunity. Extracts made up of raw thymus from animals are sometimes used to boost the human immune system. The adrenal glands are endocrine glands located above the kidneys that secrete hormones that are involved in stress management. Raw adrenal extracts are sometimes used to boost adrenal function.

Uva-Ursi—An anti-bacterial herb that has been used to treat recurrent urinary tract and other bacterial infections.

Xenoestrogens—Estrogens that are from sources outside of the body that are derived from synthetic and natural sources that interfere with normal estrogen activity.

Yeast Overgrowth/Candida—Candida is a fungus that causes yeast infection, especially in the mouth and vagina. It can also be found in the blood and spread to other organs like the intestines where it can cause symptoms such as gas, bloating, irritable bowel, fatigue, and memory and concentration problems. There are different strains of Candida, the most pervasive being Candida Albicans.

Selected References

CHAPTER 2

Bland, Jeffrey, PhD. "Nutrigenomic Modulation of Inflammatory Disorders," Metagenics Educational Program, 2004.

Chen, Mitchell, D.O., PhD. "Nutraceutical Approaches to Coronary Artery Disease," *Nutri News*, March/April 2002.

Disascio et al. "Antioxidant Defense Systems: The Carotenoids, Tocopherols and Thiols," *Am J Clin Nutr.*, 53:199s-200s.

Djoss, EL, et al. "Dietary Linolenic Acid and Carotid Atherosclerosis," The Natural Heart, Lung and Blood Institute Family Heart Study. *Am J Clin Nutr.*, 2003, 77(4) 819-25.

Eades, Michael & Mary, M.D.'s, *Protein Power,* (New York: Bantam Books, 1996).

Everson, G.T., et al. "Effects of Psyllium Hydrophilic Mucillioid on LDL-Cholesterol and Bile Acid Synthesis in Hypercholesterolemic Men," *J Lipid Res.*, 1992; 33: 1183-1192.

Hu, F.B., et al. "Fish and Long-Chain Omega-3 Fatty Acid Intake and Risk of Coronary Heart Disease and Total Mortality in Diabetic Women," *Circulation*, 2003;107 (14) 1852-7.

Langsjoen, PH, Langsjoen, AM. "Overview of the Uses of CoQ10 in Cardiovascular Disease," *Biofactors,* 1999; 9 (2-4):273-84.

Mensink, R.P., Katan, M.B. "Effects of Dietary Fatty Acids on Serum Lipids and Lipoproteins: A meta-analysis of 27 Trials," *Arterioscler Thromb.* 1992, 12: 911-919.

Miller, Alan L., N.D. "Cardiovascular Disease-Toward a Unified Approach," *Alternative Medicine Review,* Volume 1:3, 132-144.

"Natural Management of Abnormal Blood Lipids," *Designs For Health Weekly*, June, 2003.

Park, Alice. "What can You Do?" Time Magazine, February, 2004.

Pi-Sonyer, M.D. "The New Guidelines, Impacts of Obesity on Health," *Obesity from Pediatrics to Geriatrics: The problems/The solutions,* Columbia University, November, 2003.

Tran M.T., et al. "Role of Coenzyme Q10 in Chronic Heart Failure, Angina and Hypertension," *Pharmacotherapy,* July 2001; 21(7: 797-806).

CHAPTER 3

Brigelius-Flohe, R., Traber, MG. "Vitamin E: Function and Metabolism," *FASEB J.* 13:1145-1155, 1999.

Cooney, Beth. "Meditating On the Empty Cradle," *The Advocate Health & Science,* April 27, 1999.

Deckelbaum, Richard J, M.D. "Under-Appreciated Dangers: Effect of Pre-Pregnancy Obesity on Maternal and Infant Outcomes," *Obesity from pediatrics to Geriatrics: The Problems/The Solutions,* Columbia University, November 15, 2003.

Evans, Joel M.D. and Bland, Jeffery, PhD. "Natural Solutions for Managing Menopause," Metagenics Seminar, November, 2003.

Fugh-Berman, Adriane, M.D. And Kronenberg, Fredi, PhD. "Complementary and Alternative Medicine in Reproductive-aged Women: A review of Randomized Controlled Trials," *Reproductive Toxicology:* 17 (2003) 137-152.

Gittleman, Ann Louise, PhD. *Before the Change.* (San Francisco: Harper Collins Publishers, 1998).

Gittleman, Ann Louise, PhD. *Super Nutrition for Menopause.* Avery, 1998.

"If Not Hormone Therapy for Hot Flashes, Then What?" *Tufts University Health And Nutrition Letter,* March 2001.

Kahn, Sherry, M.P.H. "Sow the Seeds of Pregnancy," *Great Life,* October, 2001.

Kronenberg, Fredi, PhD. and Fugh-Berman, Adriane, M.D. "Complimentary and Alternative Medicine for Menopausal Symptoms: A Review of Randomized, Controlled Trials." *Ann Intern Med.*, 2002; 137: 805-813.

"Lack Of Vitamin B12 Linked to Repeat Miscarriage," Reuters Health, 2001.

London, R.S., et al. "The Effect of Alpha-Tocopherol on Premenstrual Symptomatology: a Double Blind Study." *J Am Coll Nutr.* 2(2): 115-122, 1983.

Northrop, Christiane, M.D. *The Wisdom of Menopause.* (New York: Bantam Books, 2003).

Simon, Renee A, M.S., C.N.S. "Natural Approaches to Infertility & Other Problems," *Resolve of Fairfield County, Inc.*, Winter, 1999/2000.

Stein, Robert. "Antibiotics May Raise Risk for Breast Cancer," *The Washington Post* (February 17, 2004).

Turner, Lisa "Boost Your fertility," *Great life*, February 2000.

CHAPTER 4

"Immune Health Guide." Immuno Laboratories, Inc., Florida.

Liska, Deann J., PhD. And Lukaczer, Dan, ND "Gut Dysfunction and Chronic Disease: The Benefits of Applying the 4R GI Restoration Program," *Applied Nutritional Science Reports*, 2001.

Plummer, Nigel, M.D. "Probiotics and Prebiotics-More than Just a Gut Feeling," Boulderfest Conference, 2004.

Rouse, James, N.D. "Nutritional Management of Irritable Bowel Syndrome," *Applied Nutritional Science Reports*, 2001.

Wilson, Jay, D.C. "Celiac Disease and Gluten Intolerance," Boulderfest, Conference, 2004.

CHAPTER 5

Amen, Daniel, M.D. *Healing A.D.D.* (New York: Berkley Books, 2001).

Bach Flower Essences for the Family. (Great Britain: Wigmore Publications Ltd. 1993).

Bell, Rachel and Peiper, Howard. *The A.D.D. and A.D.H.D. Diet.* (Safe Goods/New Century Publishing, 2000).

Brady, David, D.C., CCN, N.D. "Food Allergy & Sensitivity Lecture," 2004.

Crook, William, M.D. *Solving the Puzzle of Your Hard-To-Raise-Child.* (Tennessee: Professional Books, 1987).

Edelson, Stephen, M.D. *Conquering Autism.* (New York: Kensington Publishing Corp., 2003.

Geier & Geier, "Thimerosal In Childhood Vaccines, Neurodevelopmental Disorders, and Heart Disease in the United States," *J. Amer. Physicians & Surgeons* V8, #1, p6-11, 2003.

Harik-Khan, RI, et al. "Serum Vitamin Levels and the Risk of Asthma in Children", *Am J Epidemiol.* 2004; 159(4); 351-7.

Holmes, Amy, M.D., Blaxill, M. and Haley, C. "Mercury Birth Hair Levels vs. Amalgam Fillings in Autistic and Control Groups," *Int. J. of Toxicology* v22, In press, 2003.

Kidd, Parris, PhD. "A.D.H.D. in Children: Rationale for Its Integrative Management," *Alternative Medicine Review*, Volume 5, Number 5, 2000, V02-4281.

Klinghardt, Dietrich, MD., PhD. "Chronic Illness and Mercury Toxicity," Boulder fest Conference, 2004.

Liska, Deann J, PhD. and Lukaczer, Dan, N.D. "Gut Dysfunction and Chronic Disease: The Benefits of Applying the 4R. GI Restoration Program," *Applied Nutritional Science Reports*, 2001.

Marohn, Stephanie. *The Natural medicine Guide to Autism.* (Virginia: Hampton Roads Publishing Company, Inc, 2002).

McDonnell, Maureen, BS, RN. "Ten Tips for Keeping Our Children Healthy," Staff Training for the DAN! Protocol, TLC Seminars, 2000.

Plummer, Nigel, M.D. "Probiotics and Prebiotics-More than just a Gut Feeling," Boulderfest Conference, 2004.

Richardson, AJ, Puri BK. "A Randomized Double Blind, Placebo-Controlled Study of the Effects of Supplementation with Highly Unsaturated Fatty Acids on A.D.H.D. related Symptoms in Children with Specific Learning Difficulties," *Prog Neuropsychopharmacol Biol Psychiatry,*. 2002 Feb; 26(2) 233-9.

Reed, Rene, D.C., D.A. B.C.O. "Does What you Eat Make You Ill?," *Total Health for Longevity,* 22(6) 52-53.

Rountree, Robert. M.D., "Proven Therapeutic Benefits Of High Quality Probiotics," *Applied Nutritional Science Reports*, 2002.

CHAPTER 6

Baker, Sidney MacDonald. *Detoxification & Healing* (Connecticut: Keats Publishing, Inc., 1997).

Murray, Michael, N.D., and Pizzorno, Joseph, N.D. *Encyclopedia Of Natural Medicine*, (California: Prima Health, 1998).

CHAPTER 7

Bendich, A. "Carotenoids and the Immune Response." *J. Nutr.,* 1989; 119: 112-115.

Di Masco, et al. "Antioxidant Defense Systems: The Carotenoids, Tocopherols & Thiols." *Am. J. Clin. Nutr.,* 53: 194S-200S.

Lee, Roberta, M.D. "Medical Uses of Chocolate." *Botanical medicine in Modern Clinical Practice,* Columbia University, 2004.

Rubin, Bruce, Stress, Immune Function & Health: The Connection. Wiley-Liss (February, 1999).

Vedantam, Shaker. "Study finds Link Between Emotions, Immune System," *The Washington Post.* (January 20, 2004);

CHAPTER 8

Agatson, Arthur, M.D. *The South Beach Diet.* (Emmaus, Penn.: Rodale, 2003).
Atkins, Robert, M.D. *Dr. Atkins New Diet Revolution.* (New York: Avon Books, 2002).
DeNoon, Daniel. "Many 'Healthy Foods' Full of Unlabeled Trans Fats," *Webmed Medical News,* February 10, 2003.
Gittleman, Ann Louise, M.S., C.N.S. *Eat fat, Lose Weight.* (Illinois: Keats Publishing, 1999).
Hsu–Leblanc, Elisabeth. "Farmed vs. Wild Caught," *Taste for Life,* March, 2004.
Lemonick, Michael "Eat Your Heart Out," *Time,* July 19, 1999.
Sears, Barry. *The Zone:* (New York: Harper Collins Books, 1995).
Serafina, M., R. Bugianesei, et al. "Plasma Antioxidants from Chocolate," *Nature* 424.6952 (2004) 1013.
"The Details: Fat & Fatty Acids." The American Heart Association Website.
Wolcott, William and Fahey, Trish. *The Metabolic Typing Diet* (New York: Broadway Books, 2002).
Yanovski, S. "Sugar and Fat: Cravings and Aversions," *Journal Of Nutrition* 133.3 (2003); 835s-7s.

CHAPTER 9

Brown, Richard, M.D. and Gerbarg, Patricia, M.D. *The Rhodiola Revolution,* Rodale, 2004
Carper, Jean. *Stop Aging Now,* (New York: Harper Collins Publishers, Inc., 1995).

Carper, Jean, *Miracle Cures*, (New York: Harper Collins Books, 1997).
La Valle, James, R.Ph., C.C.N., N.D. *Cracking The Metabolic Code.* (New Jersey: Basic Health Publications, Inc., 2004).

CHAPTER 11

Mills, James Willard, PhD. *Coping with Stress.* (New York: John Wiley & Sons, Inc., 1982).
Shames, Richard, M.D. "Nutritional Management of Stress–Induced Dysfunction," *Advanced Nutrition Publications, Inc.*, 2002.

Resources

This section lists the vitamin companies and labs that I have used successfully in my practice and feel most comfortable with. It also provides information on website links that you might find helpful.

Supplement Companies

These companies have pharmaceutical grade products with excellent manufacturing and product quality controls. Most of these companies work directly with nutritionists. If you want to order products from any of these companies you can give them my name if you are not working with another nutritionist.

Allergy Research Group

Distributed by: Moss Nutrition
2 Bay Road, Suite 102
Hadley, Ma 01035
Tel: 800 851 5444, Fax: 413 587 0331
Mossnutrition.com

Dr. Stephen A.Levine, Ph.D founded this company in 1979. Dr. Levine was the first to introduce products free of all common allergens and since then his company has expanded their products based on recent research outcomes.

Ameriden International, LLC

P.O. Box 1870
Fallbrook, Ca 92088

Tel: 760 728 0747, Fax: 760 728 0608 ameriden.com

Ameriden offers naturally derived products among which Rosavin (Rhodiola rosea) is of special interest. This supplement aids in improvement of memory, mental, and physical performance as well as maintaining energy levels.

Biogenesis Nutraceuticals. Inc

Distributed by: Moss Nutrition
2 Bay Road, Suite 102
Hadley Ma 01035
Tel: 800 851 5444, Fax: 413 587 0331
mossnutrition.com

Biogenesis has a wide variety of products. They are licensed as a food, nutritional and OTC drug manufacturer. Their products are tested through HPLC, gas chromatography, mass spectrometry atomic absorption and flame emission spectrophotometry. Biogenesis offers the product Biofocus that was mentioned in the children's section of the book. This product is very effective for ADHD and other disorders where focus and attention are problems.

Crayhon Research, Inc.

5355 Capital Court # 101
Reno, NV 89502
Tel: 877 CRAYHON
CrayhonResearch.com

Crayhon Research designs and creates high quality supplements that have clinical efficacy using the latest research available. They use GMP standards and raw ingredients that come from Europe and the USA that are top quality. One of their primary goals is to educate health care practitioners on the latest findings in clinical nutrition.

Designs for Health

2 North Road
East Windsor, CT 06088
Tel: 800 847 8302, Fax: 860627 0661
designsforhealth.com
Also distributed by Moss Nutrition, see above

Designs for Health offers many therapeutic nutrients which are research driven and synergistically formulated. They are also an educational company providing weekly teleconference clinical rounds and monthly nutritional roundtables for practitioners.

Kirkman Laboratories

6400 SW Rosewood Street
Lake Oswego, Oregon 97035
Tel: 800 245 8282, Fax: 503 6682 0838
Kirkmanlabs.com, kirkman @kirkmanlabs.com

This company was established in 1949 and offers a wide range of nutritional supplements designed for people with sensitivities and special needs i.e. children with developmental disorders.

Metagenics

100 Avenida La Pata
San Clemente, Ca 92673
Tel: 800 692 9400
metagenics.com

Metagenics manufactures nutraceutical products designed to enhance positive genetic expression and improve health. They utilize new technology to produce formulations that manifest a "multifunctional synergy."

Nordic Naturals

Distributed by: Moss Nutrition
2 Bay Road, Suite 102
Hadley, Ma 01035
Tel: 800 851 5444, Fax: 413 587 0331
mossnutrition.com

This company offers a varied range of Omega 3 fatty acids with different natural fruit flavors that are especially helpful for children. Their products have all been carefully processed to be free of heavy metals and low in oxidation levels.

Pharmax, LLC

1239 120th Ave NE, Suite B
Bellevue, WA 98005
Tel: 425/467.8054; 800/538.8274
Fax: 425/467.9112
hq@pharmaxllc.com

Pharmax was established in 2002 and is directed by Dr. Nigel Plummer in the UK. Dr. Plummer has been involved in extensive research on probiotics, fatty acids, and plant antimicrobials. Pharmax offers a wide range of supplements which reflect a scientific and logical approach.

Shaklee Corporation

4747 Willow Road
Pleasanton, Ca 94588
800 742.5533
Shaklee.com

Dr. Forrest C. Shaklee and his two sons founded this Company in 1956. The company's mission has been to develop natural supplements that are free of environmental pollutants, pesticides, lead, arsenic, organic solvents, residues and synthetics materials. This company manufactures the glucose regulation complex product that was mentioned earlier. In addition to nutritional supplements, Shaklee offers a full line of chemical free cleaning, laundry and personal care products, as well as water and air purification systems. You need to be a member to order through the 800 phone number or website. If you do not have a Shaklee distributor to help you, use my member number: DA56937DS or my website www.totalwellnessnutrition.com.

Laboratories

Analytical Research labs, Inc.

2225 West Alice Avenue
Phoenix, Arizona 85021
Tel: 602 995-1580
www.arltma.com

This company analyzes tissue mineral content through hair analysis. Hair analysis is one of the diagnostic tools used by many health practitioners to identify the body's rate of metabolism, imbalances in glandular systems, toxic metals, and mineral deficiencies/excesses.

Cell Science Systems, Ltd. Corp

1239 E. Newport Center Dr., Suite 101
Deerfield Beach, FL., 33442
Tel: 954 923 2990/800 881 2685, Fax: 954 923 2707
Alcat.com

CSS offers ALCAT testing which is a registered trademark of Cell Science Systems, Ltd. Corp. The ALCAT test determines sensitivities or delayed adverse reactions to over 100 foods and additives. A food rotation plan based on the test result is also provided to patients. This test utilizes whole blood, as opposed to just serum. Rather than only checking for IgG antibodies formed in response to particular food proteins, it actually analyzes cellular changes that occur to leukocytes and platelets when they are exposed to challenge substances. The test utilizes significantly modified proprietary Coulter cell analyzer technology, which can accurately and electronically detect minute changes in WBC morphology, platelet aggregation, and plasma protein alterations that can result from intolerance or allergy phenomena. This methodology can detect sensitive responses on multiple pathways, not just IgG.

Great Smokies Diagnostic Laboratory

63 Zillicoa Street
Asheville, NC 28800
800 522 4762
cs@gsdl.com

This laboratory specializes in doing comprehensive digestive stool analysis. They also do a variety of other functional assessments for patients including saliva hormone tests, amino and fatty acid analysis, and urine and hair analysis for toxic metals.

Immuno laboratories Inc.

1620 West Oakland Park Blvd.
Fort Lauderdale, Florida 33311
Tel: 800 231 9197/954 486 4500
Fax: 954 739 6563
www. Immunolabs.com

This laboratory offers tests using the Rebello method of optimiza-tion-a scientific series of techniques and procedures developed by the director, John Rebello, PhD. This lab performs comprehensive food allergy/sensitivity tests and utilizes a process named "Bloodprint" which is their registered trademark.

NeuroScience Laboratory

15 Loop Rd. #106
Arden, NC 28704
Tel: 866 651 0250, Fax: 828 651 0379
Neuroscienceinc.com

Neuroscience specializes in the assessment and connection of neu-rotransmitters. Medical research has shown that many problems associ-ated with today's fast-paced lifestyle can be linked to an imbalance in neurotransmitters and hormone levels. They have pioneered a unique systematic approach to understanding, monitoring and optimizing neurotransmitter levels and utilizing the result through urine testing.

Rosmed

809 8th St. Suite 7
Miami Beach, Florida 33139
Tel: 305 864 3828, Fax: 305 864 3606
DrInstitute@bellsouth.net

This German based lab specializes in comprehensive stool analysis called *Whole health GI Assessment Panel*. This test offers markers which include: stool *histamine* (for food intolerance and allergy), *pmn-granulocyte-elastase* (for acute inflammation), *antitrypsin* (for chronic inflammation), *lactoferrin* (for differentiation between inflammation and irritable bowel), *pancreatic elastase*s for pancreatic function, microscopic markers for meat and vegetable fibers, digestive residues (*fat, protein, sugar, fiber, water*) and digestive enzymes (*bile acids*). Stool flora assessment includes all beneficial and burdening bacteria and yeasts, measured in absolute *colony-forming-units* per gram stool.

The Great Plains Laboratory

11813 W 77th Street
Lenexa, KS 66214
Tel: 913 341 8949, Fax: 913 341 6207
Greatplainslaborary.com
Gpl4u@aol.com

This laboratory specializes in Autism, PDD, ADHD and related disorders. The director Dr. Shaw, father of an autistic child actively employs parents of children with autism on his staff to ensure representation of views and concerns. Their most popular test is the Organic Acid urine profile.

York Nutritional Laboratories Inc.

2700 North 29th Ave., Suite 205
Hollywood, Florida 33020
Tel: 888 751-3388
info@yorkallergyusa.com

This laboratory is the developer of *food*SCAN tm, a "finger stick" IgG Elisa food intolerance test kit that is performed at home. This test has been validated by multiple independent studies and is especially good for children who have difficulty getting their blood drawn.

Websites

www.totalwellnessnutrition.com - This is my official website. You can contact me to set up a phone or in person consultation or to sign up for my free electronic newsletter and recipes. There is also more information on ordering products that were mentioned in the book, as well as articles, interviews, and patient testimonials.

www.rhodeolarosea.org - An excellent source of information and research on Rhodeola rosea.

Organizations

Art of Living-Provides information on yoga and breathing courses available throughout the United States and the world. - www.artofliving.org
Autism Research Institute - www.autismwebsite.com/ari/
Center for Science in the public interest - www.cspinet.org
Dietary Supplement Information Bureau - www.supplementinfo.org
Herb Research Foundation - www.herbs.org
Medline Abstract Search - www.ncbi.nlm.nih.gov/pubmed
National Center for Complimentary and Alternative Medicine (NCCAM) - www.nccam.nih.gov
Resolve-National Fertility Organization - www.resolve.org

Special Diets

Gluten Free Sites:

www.glutensolutions.com

www.glutenfree.com
www.glutenfreemall.com
www.missroben.com
www.glutino.com

Specific Carbohydrate Diet - www.scdiet.org
The Feingold Program - www.feingold.org

Index

978-0-595-34891-6
0-595-34891-2

Printed in the United States
42669LVS00004B/157